General Practice and Ethics

With the reorganization of general practice and the NHS, GPs now face many new and distinctive ethical dilemmas in their practice. Pressures on resources coupled with an increasing concern to evaluate the outcomes of health care mean that GPs now have additional responsibilities, responsibilities which could conflict with the primary objective of caring for the individual patient.

General Practice and Ethics explores the ethical issues that are encountered by GPs in their everyday practice, addressing two central themes: the uncertainty of outcomes and effectiveness in general practice and the changing pattern of general practitioners' responsibilities. Among the topics examined are:

- the ethical implications of the use of evidence-based medicine in general practice
- consent, autonomy and confidentiality in general practice
- the history of patient-centredness
- the ethics of prescribing
- research ethics in general practice

General Practice and Ethics presents a topical and comprehensive analysis of the kinds of ethical dilemmas faced by GPs on a daily basis which will be useful to practitioners and students alike.

Christopher Dowrick is Professor of Primary Medical Care at the University of Liverpool and a general practitioner in North Liverpool.
Lucy Frith is Lecturer in Health Care Ethics at the University of Liverpool. She is the editor of *Midwifery Ethics: A Multi-disciplinary approach* (1996).

Professional Ethics

General editor: Ruth Chadwick

Centre for Applied Ethics, University of Wales College of Cardiff

Professionalism is a subject of interest to academics, the general public and would-be professional groups. Traditional ideas of professions and professional conduct have been challenged by recent social, political and technological changes. One result has been the development for almost every profession of an ethical code of conduct which attempts to formalize its values and standards. These codes of conduct raise a number of questions about the status of a 'profession' and the consequent moral implications for behaviour.

This series, edited from the Centre for Applied Ethics in Cardiff, seeks to examine these questions both critically and constructively. Individual volumes will consider issues relevant to particular professions, including nursing, genetics counselling and law. Other volumes will address issues relevant to all professional groups such as the function and value of a code of ethics and the demands of confidentiality.

Also available in the series:

Current Issues in Business Ethics
Edited by Peter W.F. Davies

Ethical Issues in Accounting
Edited by Catherine Crowthorpe and John Blake

Ethical Issues in Nursing
Edited by Geoffrey Hunt

Ethical Issues in Social Work
Edited by Richard Hugman and David Smith

Ethics and Community in the Health Care Professions
Edited by Mike Parker

Ethics and Values in Health Care Management
Edited by Souzy Dracopoulou

Genetic Counselling
Edited by Angus Clarke

The Ground of Professional Ethics
Daryl Koehn

The Ethics of Bankruptcy
Jukka Kilpi

Food Ethics
Edited by Ben Mepham

General Practice and Ethics

Uncertainty and responsibility

Edited by
Christopher Dowrick and
Lucy Frith

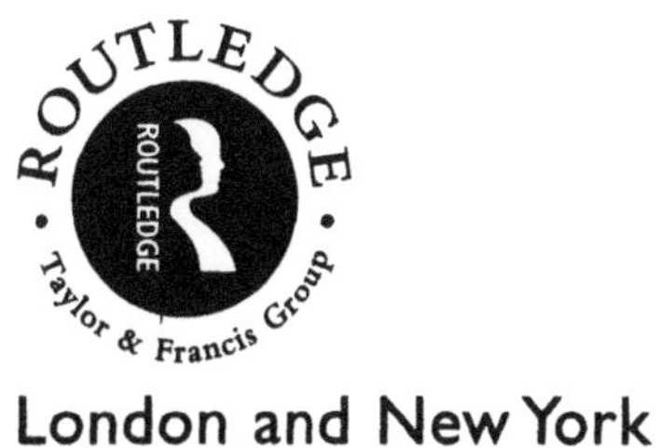

London and New York

First published 1999
by Routledge
2 Park Square, Milton Park, Abingdon, Oxon, OX14 4RN

Simultaneously published in the USA and Canada
by Routledge
29 West 35th Street, New York, NY 10001

Routledge is an imprint of the Taylor & Francis Group

Transferred to Digital Printing 2004

Typeset in Times New Roman by
Ponting–Green Publishing Services, Chesham, Bucks

British Library Cataloguing in Publication Data
A catalogue record for this book is available from the British Library

Library of Congress Cataloging in Publication Data
General practice and ethics / edited by Christopher Dowrick and Lucy Frith
p. cm. — (Professional ethics)
Includes bibliographical references and index.
1. Physicians (General practice)—Professional ethics. 2. Primary care (Medicine)—Moral and ethical aspects. 3. Evidence-based medicine—Moral and ethical aspects. 4. Medical ethics.
I. Dowrick, Christopher. II. Frith, Lucy. III. Series.
R725.5.G46 1999
174'.2—dc21 98–38318

ISBN 0–415–16498–2 (hbk)
ISBN 0–415–16499–0 (pbk)

Contents

Notes on contributors

Colin Bradley is Professor of General Practice and Head of Department at University College Cork, Ireland. His research on general practitioners' prescribing dilemmas highlighted the fact that many prescribing difficulties are really ethical problems. He continues to be involved in research on doctor–patient communication which will address some of the ethical dimensions of prescribing. He has also taught medical ethics at the University of Birmingham Medical School.

Angus Dawson is a philosopher who teaches health care ethics at the University of Liverpool. He is currently completing his PhD, which is a consideration of the methodological foundations of applied ethics.

Christopher Dowrick was a historian, social worker and psychotherapist before turning to medicine. He is now Professor of Primary Medical Care at the University of Liverpool and a general practitioner in North Liverpool. His main academic interests are in doctor–patient relationships and in the management of mental health in primary care.

Len Doyal is Professor of Medical Ethics at St Bartholomew's and the Royal London School of Medicine and Dentistry, Queen Mary and Westfield College, University of London. He is also an Honorary Consultant to the Royal Hospital's Trust. Professor Doyal's most recent book is *A Theory of Human Needs* (with Ian Gough). He writes widely on ethico-legal issues applied to medicine and dentistry.

Lucy Frith is a philosopher who specializes in health care ethics and is Lecturer in Health Care Ethics at the University of Liverpool. She is a fellow of the Institute of Law, Medicine and Bioethics. Her research interests include women's health and midwifery and the ethical aspects of the evidence-based medicine and effectiveness debate in health care.

Roger Higgs is a general practitioner in South London and Professor and Head of the Department of General Practice and Primary Care at King's College School of Medicine and Dentistry in London. He has been Case Conference Editor of the *Journal of Medical Ethics*, and has published widely in the field, including *The New Dictionary of Medical Ethics* with Anthony Pinching and Kenneth Boyd.

Roger Jones is Wolfson Professor of General Practice at Guy's, King's and St Thomas's School of Medicine, London. He has a long-standing interest in research in primary care and in the links between research findings and professional behavioural change. He is editor of *Family Practice*, an international journal of primary health care.

Jean McHale is Senior Lecturer in Law, Faculty of Law, University of Manchester and also a director of the Centre for Social Ethics and Policy in the University of Manchester.

Carl May is Senior Research Fellow in Medical Sociology in the Department of General Practice, University of Manchester. He has researched and published widely on professional–patient interaction in nursing, general practice and genetic counselling.

Nicola Mead read biology and philosophy at the University of Manchester before joining the staff of the National Primary Care Research and Development Centre, where she is now a Research Associate. Her current work is on patient empowerment and quality in the consultation.

Sam Smith is a general practitioner and part-time clinical lecturer at the Department of Primary Care, University of Liverpool. His interests include the doctor's relationship with 'difficult patients', counselling and psychotherapy in general practice, and postmodern philosophy.

General editor's foreword

Professional ethics is now acknowledged as a field of study in its own right. Much of its recent development has resulted from rethinking traditional medical ethics in the light of new moral problems arising out of advances in medical science and technology. Applied philosophers, ethicists and lawyers have devoted considerable energy to exploring the dilemmas emerging from modern health care practices and their effects on the practitioner–patient relationship.

It is fair to say, however, that the ethical issues that arise in general practice have received less attention than, for example, those in hospital-based medicine. As the editors of this volume show, however, it is in general practice that some of the most complex issues arise, for example management of chronic illness and the establishment of relationships with whole families over time, with the possibility of conflicting obligations.

Christopher Dowrick and Lucy Frith point out that government policies regarding the emphasis on primary care, on the one hand, and the increasing focus on resource shortages, on the other, have only served to highlight the fact that general practitioners often face difficult ethical choices, arising in part out of their changing responsibilities. Responsibility forms one of the main themes of the volume. The other is uncertainty, for example in relation to outcomes and effectiveness in general practice, and how that impacts on ethical decision-making.

In so far as the volume deals with changing patterns of health care it should be of interest to all those with an interest in health care ethics, and not only to those concerned with the particular field of general practice.

The Professional Ethics series seeks to examine ethical issues in the professions and related areas both critically and constructively. Individual volumes address issues relevant to all professional groups, such as the nature of a profession. Other volumes examine issues relevant to particular professions, including those which have hitherto received little attention, such as the topic of this volume, health care management and the insurance industry.

Ruth Chadwick

Acknowledgements

We would like to thank Ruth Chadwick and Andrew Belsey for inviting us to produce this volume and the people at Routledge for their help with the editorial and production process. Nicci Jones deserves a special thank you for her invaluable contribution to the editorial and administrative side of the project. Lucy Frith would like to thank her parents, Margaret and David, and Mark Tanner for their help in proofreading the manuscript and for their general encouragement and support. Chris Dowrick would like to thank Mark Fisher for stimulating philosophical comment and Sue Martin for being there.

Introduction

BACKGROUND

The pattern of health care provision is changing in Britain, due to the increasing focus on primary care. This is exemplified by the policies of the Labour government (elected in 1997) that stipulated that the majority of health care should eventually be provided in a primary care setting. As a reflection of this trend, undergraduate medical education is now based more in the community rather than in the hospital. These changes in medical education will influence the priorities and expertise of future doctors and elevate the status of primary care medicine. These initiatives could be argued to be an illustration of a conceptual shift from a biomedical model of health to a biopsychosocial approach. Under the biomedical model the patient is seen as a diseased body part and treated accordingly, the patient's social and personal circumstances are of limited importance in the treatment regime and the hospital becomes the most appropriate place for providing health care. The biopsychosocial approach attempts to see the patient as a complete individual with biological, psychological and social elements that all impact and influence the patient's health. Primary care medicine is much better placed than hospital based care to provide this kind of medical care, operating in the community in which the patient lives and seeing the patient on a regular and long-term basis. Due to these practical and conceptual changes general practitioners have an increasingly important role in health care provision and, with this growing role, additional responsibilities.

This collection is an exploration of the ethical issues that are encountered by general practitioners in their everyday practice. The issues are considered from a variety of perspectives: general practitioners who specialize in different areas, philosophers and lawyers. The book is a collection of perspectives and viewpoints of different authors and is not a reflection of one view of general practice or one view of what is ethically acceptable. We have, however, asked the contributors to address two central themes in their chapters: the uncertainty of outcomes and effectiveness in general practice and the changing pattern of general practitioners' responsibilities. These are central themes not only for general practice and primary care but for all health care provision.

One of the most important concerns for modern health care practice is how health care is to be paid for. All medical practice now takes place in an environment of limited resources, whether it is a national health service or a privately-owned insurance led system. With this concern for the financial implications of health care provision comes an increasing concern to ensure that all treatments provided have been proved to be useful and effective. When areas for economy are being considered, it seems self-evident that those treatments that are not effective – that do not produce the results intended or good enough results – should not be provided or commissioned. Many areas of general practice are shrouded in uncertainty because patients present with a complex set of both medical and social problems. General practice is also often concerned with the management of chronic health problems, and this makes it very hard to determine the outcomes of treatments and therefore to define effectiveness in a general practice context. This raises the difficult question of what sort of treatments general practitioners should be providing and what considerations should govern these decisions so that they are taken ethically.

General practitioners, just like all health care professionals, have to work in this environment of concern for the wider financial implications of their decisions. No longer is the individual patient the only focus of concern; the general practitioner has to take into consideration the implications of treatment decisions for their practice, the health authority and ultimately the health service as a whole. Hence, these additional responsibilities could potentially conflict with the primary objective of caring for the individual patient. General practitioners need some way of resolving these conflicts ethically so that, ultimately, patient care does not suffer. These changes in the organization of health care and particularly primary care mean that general practitioners need to be aware of the ethical dimension of their practice and ethical literature should reflect these distinctive concerns.

ETHICS AND GENERAL PRACTICE

The purpose of this introduction is not to give a detailed or comprehensive account of what ethics is or an introduction to ethical theory, but we thought it would be useful to briefly consider the approach that is taken in this collection and the areas of ethical reasoning that are addressed.

Very broadly, ethics can be defined as the study of the moral aspects of our lives and can cover a wide range of theoretical and practical areas. This collection is largely concerned with the application of ethical reasoning to general practice to determine the acceptability of actions or policies.

The important area of ethics for the purposes of this collection is normative ethics.[1] Normative ethics is concerned with establishing norms of conduct, and developing ethical theories or principles that can govern decision making and practice. Hence, normative ethics evaluates the moral acceptability of a decision or a course of action. The application of normative theories or principles to actual situations, such as medicine or public policy, is called applied ethics, i.e. the attempt to apply these theoretical deliberations and come to some conclusions on the morality of particular situations.

In the area of medicine one particular normative approach to solving ethical dilemmas has become very popular: the four principles of health care ethics. The four principles approach, as it has been called, is defended by such authors as Gillon (1985) and Beauchamp and Childress (1994). This approach sets out four principles – respect for autonomy, beneficence, minimizing harm and justice – that can be applied to ethical dilemmas in an attempt to determine what is the right course of action. We will give a brief outline of these four principles.

Autonomy is the doctrine that the individual human will is or ought to be governed by its own principles and laws. It is closely related to concepts of self-determination and personal freedom. It can have both a passive and an active component. In its passive sense it implies freedom from external control or influence. In its active sense it contains the assumption of a capacity for independent action. The most concrete way patient autonomy is respected in medical practice is in obtaining consent for medical procedures, which encapsulates the belief that it is the patient who, ultimately, should make the choice over what procedures to undergo without undue coercion from the medical practitioner.

Beneficence refers to the act of doing good. It is a stronger word than benevolence (wishing good), since it assumes action. It includes preventing harm, removing harm and actively promoting good. 'The *principle of beneficence* refers to a moral obligation to act for the benefit of others' (Beauchamp and Childress,1994: 260). Hence it covers all possible aspects of medical activity, from disease prevention through cancer surgery to advanced pharmacotherapeutics. Health care professionals have an actual duty to do good for their patients which is often expressed as a duty of care and describes the special relationship that doctors have with their patients. This duty is more extensive than the average person's duties as, in our personal lives, we are under no obligation to act as good Samaritans to others, just refrain from harming them, unless we are in some form of special relationship with them such as parent and child.

The duty to minimize harm, or non-maleficence, is historically rendered in the Latin phrase *primum non nocere*, or 'first do no harm'. As Gillon says, 'Thus the traditional Hippocratic moral obligation of medicine is to provide net medical benefit to patients with minimal harm – that is, beneficence with non-maleficence' (1985: 185). The principle of non-maleficence is often seen as the other side of the beneficence coin and, as Gillon says, the two principles are closely related as doing good often implies not harming.

Justice is a difficult principle to define, but it is broadly fair, equitable and appropriate treatment. It implies freedom from discrimination or dishonesty and impartiality. It is often restated as 'distributive justice', or the determination of rights, and stipulates that the benefits and burdens of society should be distributed fairly in accordance with a particular conception of what are considered to be similarly deserving cases. This is the formal principle of justice, that equals should be treated equally. The difficult question here is how is equality to be defined? Should it mean equal wealth? Equal intelligence? Equal need? Or equal deservingness? In health care equal intelligence does not seem a just way of distributing health care resources, but an argument can be made that it is a just way of distributing places at universities. Equal need appears to be a better definition of equality to base the just distribution of health care resource upon, but this is not without problems, as someone may greatly need health care but it would not prolong their life or they might not 'deserve it' by having contributed to their own ill health. In general practice principles of justice are particularly relevant, for example, when considering the debate about whether fund holding has created a 'two tier' health care system, or whether limited resources should be deployed in coronary artery bypass grafting or the management of incontinence.

To give a simple example of the application of the four principles of health care ethics approach: a patient comes into a surgery, violent and angry, shouting at the staff and those in the waiting room and threatening to harm himself. This patient has a history of self-abuse and at times this abuse has nearly proved fatal. You attempt to calm the patient, but he says that he wants to be allowed to leave and says that he will try and kill himself when he gets home. What should the general practitioner do? In this situation using the four principles approach, the GP would have to weigh up respecting the patient's autonomy by allowing him to go home or trying to promote beneficence for the patient by instigating some form of restraint of the patient.

The main difficulty with applying the four principles in practice is, as illustrated by the example above, what course of action should we take if two or more of the principles conflict? What do we do if doing good for a patient involves restricting his autonomy? Which principle should take precedence? The four principles are only *prima facie* obligations, that is the obligations must be followed unless they conflict with another obligation that is equal or stronger, giving us no clear guidance on which principle should take precedence. This is often seen as the main criticism of the four principle approach – that it gives no guidance on action when two or more of the principles conflict. Thus, this requires us to think about the relative weight of the principles and determine which one we think should be considered the most important in a particular situation. There is no easy way of establishing the most important principle to follow in a particular case. Often it is argued that patient autonomy should take precedence, as freedom of action is seen as an unqualified good in our society and any measures that limit people's freedom, even if it is for their own good, are seen as unwarranted. There has been a move away from paternalism in medicine, which limits the patients' autonomy for their own good, and this is reflected by the increasing concern that patients give informed consent to treatments. Patient centred care is becoming a key principle in modern medical practice. However, some argue we have swung too far the other way in allowing such unfettered patient autonomy and that it threatens doctors' ability to do the best for their patients. Despite the questions that the four principles approach leave unanswered, the approach can indicate elements that should be brought to bear on a situation and hence can provide broad guidance if not definitive answers to ethical dilemmas.

The four principles of health care ethics is a recurrent theme throughout the book. Colin Bradley, for example, considers the application of the four principles to the ethics of prescribing and argues that the technical requirements of rational prescribing mirror these four principles. Roger Jones examines how the four principles can be regarded as 'cardinal duties' that apply with equal force to medical research. However, this is not to say that the four principles are unquestionably accepted by all the contributing authors. Len Doyal examines the limitations of this 'standard' view of medical ethics and analyses why it is primarily associated with acute care in hospital. Doyal concludes by suggesting that the standard view may distract attention from the socio-economic circumstances of patients in ways which can make it inconsistent with the very moral goals it advocates. Sam Smith outlines a postmodernist approach to ethics which dispenses with the notion of such abstract principles. Thus, this collection is both an attempt to see how the four principles can be applied to health care practice and a critical examination of such attempts.

AN OUTLINE OF THE COLLECTION

The book is divided into two parts. The first part considers general ethical and philosophical themes and the second part examines particular topics of importance to general practitioners. It is not possible to cover the entire spectrum of ethical issues relevant to general practice, rather we have concentrated on what we consider to be key themes and exemplary topics. However, we believe that we have provided enough information, and asked sufficiently pertinent questions, to provoke our readers into developing their own ethical perspectives on the issues which we raise and the many other issues that we have not had space to cover.

Part I: Themes

This section considers the general themes of the problems of making ethical decisions in conditions of considerable uncertainty and the tensions between the general practitioner's responsibility to both the individual patient and the wider community.

In the first chapter, Christopher Dowrick sets out to explore the uncomfortable juxtaposition of uncertainty and responsibility which lies at the heart of general practice. He describes the various levels of uncertainty which exist in ordinary general practice, and proposes a set of pragmatic strategies which doctors can use to reduce their sense of uncertainty on the one hand and maintain their sense of responsibility on the other. He then deploys concepts drawn from logic – in particular probability theory and decision analysis – to guide decision making in areas of diagnosis and management. In situations of unresolved conflict, particularly if there are conflicting value systems, he suggests that Levi's 'weighted average principle' may offer useful guidance. He suggests that the tension between uncertainty and responsibility can ultimately be a motivating force for general practitioners.

Lucy Frith then examines the ethical issues underpinning the current orthodoxy of evidence-based medicine (EBM). The aim of the chapter is to consider how medical evidence is employed in practice and how it affects clinical decision making. EBM attempts to make clinical decision making 'better', that is more scientific and less based on individual opinion. However, it will be argued that the use of EBM still involves some form of interpretation of the scientific data, which is unavoidable if the data is to be applied to treatment decisions. Although the treatment decision may be based on objective scientific data, the decision cannot be said to be an objective one, as it will be based on a value judgement about the applicability of the data to a certain situation.

In Chapter 3 Len Doyal argues that general practitioners often have to face tougher ethico-legal decisions than their hospital counterparts. The long-term relationships which they have with their patients demand the goal of promoting a patient's long-term autonomy, sometimes at the expense of respecting their autonomy in the short-term. These relationships also entail living with the moral tensions within families and coping with pressures to breach confidentiality. To help general practitioners to address these ethical problems they need more opportunity for collective discussion. It must also be remembered that medical ethics and moral character should not be divorced from attempts to improve the living and working conditions of patients, since to do so would undermine the goals of good general practice and the moral principles which inform it.

In Chapter 4 Jean McHale examines the problems surrounding maintaining patient confidentiality in everyday general practice. She describes the many situations in which disclosure of information is possible (with and without the patient's consent), including insurance claims, public interest cases, children and incompetent adults. She raises questions about confidentiality within the surgery, with respect to support staff and to sick doctors, and discusses the dilemmas arising from data protection. In practice she argues that the doctor has very considerable – and uncomfortable – powers of discretion and disclosure which depend ultimately on his or her own ethical position.

In Chapter 5 Carl May and Nicola Mead critically examine the history of the 'patient-as-person' as set out in recent accounts which suggest that this phenomenon disappeared with the rise of scientific medicine in the nineteenthth century and was only rediscovered in the second quarter of this century. They see the recent growth of 'biopsychosocial' medicine as an attempt to recapture this lost world of medical practice, and a recognition of the complex ecology of illness and disease. Contemporary medicine is awash with ideas about the patient-as-person. Enablement, empowerment, negotiation and patient-centredness form vital parts of a professional vocabulary. In general practice, especially, the patient-as-person is given enormous significance as a partner in the often complex negotiations that take place in the consultation. However, they argue that the resurgence of interest in patient-centredness may demand too much from the doctor, and may paradoxically be shifting the focus of the consultation away from the development of a relationship to the achievement of a set of technical skills.

Sam Smith finds postmodern ideas both fascinating and challenging. In the context of the extremely relativistic theses of postmodernism, and its sustained assault on conceptions of truth, certainty and the self, he asks whether it is possible to develop an ethical code in general practice that is anything other than contingent. Are doctors left with the choice of holding onto an increasingly fragile sense of biomedical certainty, or conversely of attempting to construct an ethics without foundations from a self without foundations? He counters these perspectives with two key notions drawn from Henkman and Levinas. First, that morality or ethics are constitutive of subjectivity; and second, that it is relation with the Other, in the sense of being-for rather than being-with, that our ethical position is defined and realized.

Part II: Topics

In the second section of the book we relate these themes to ethical issues and dilemmas that arise in general practice. We consider general practice prescribing, the understanding and management of depression, the expanding but complex field of advance directives and the role of research in general practice.

In Chapter 7 Colin Bradley considers the ethics of prescribing in a primary care context. His discussion of the ethics of prescribing begins from the position that the technical requirements of rational prescribing are usually backed by ethical imperatives. *Safe* prescribing is based on the principle of non-maleficence, and includes the technical aspects of drug safety, the use of unlicensed drugs, and the technical and ethical problems that arise from the unintended effects of the prescribed drugs. Beneficence requires prescribing to be *effective*: this raises questions about evidence-based medicine and health gain, and the problems of prescribing under uncertainty. Respect for autonomy requires *appropriate* prescribing, which relates to issues of informed consent, intentional non-disclosure and the role of placebos. *Economic* prescribing derives from the obligations of fairness and justice. Bradley discusses the difficulties which can arise when two or more of these imperatives are in conflict, and argues that the resolution of such difficulties usually requires ethical rather than technical judgements to be made.

In Chapter 8 Roger Higgs examines the ethical problems encountered when trying to manage depression in general practice. Higgs starts his discussion of the ethics of depression with the assumption that some certainties exist, for example that depression is diagnosable and important and that every judgement in this field is likely to have a moral component. He believes that doctors are required to pay attention as well as to offer access, to listen as well as to act, and faces us with the 'challenge of unsilencing' to improve the human predicament by giving the silent a voice. He considers the boundary of what is considered ethically acceptable to be on the move in this area and argues that to the basic four principles of ethical health care we should add the concepts of roles and responsibilities, values and virtues, perspectives and purposes. Different views of depression and mental health – whether it is the philosophical challenge of happiness or the sociological discourse of loss and challenge to identity – may be helpful in offering a properly rounded assessment of depression in primary care.

In Chapter 9 Angus Dawson examines the ethical implications of advanced directives. Dawson takes issue with the assertion that advance directives – statements by competent people about what medical treatment they do or do not want if in the future they become incompetent – is the obvious way to create ethical health care for incompetent people. He points to a strong body of empirical evidence against such directives. He doubts whether written directives can ever accurately capture what the author would want to happen, or that the decisions of a proxy can be any more than informed guesswork. It is unclear when advance directives should come into operation, or what limits should be put on the requests that can be made, and Dawson reviews the rapidly changing legal position in the UK. The philosophical issue of personal identity, what it is to be a unique individual over time, leads Dawson towards the view that advance directives should be advisory and that 'current best-interests' tests may be more a more valid basis for clinical decision making.

In the final chapter Roger Jones turns to the distinct ethical issues and dilemmas raised by the rapid increase of research activity in primary care. He stresses the need for researchers in primary care to be quite clear about their responsibilities to people in the community who have not yet sought or entered formal medical care, and to patients contacting general practitioners who are doing so in the reasonable expectation of complete confidentiality and do not regard themselves at risk of being involved in research studies. He discusses the potential for research to conflict with patient autonomy and to cause harm, in the gathering of both qualitative and quantitative data and in the dissemination of findings, and offers advice on how these ethical threats can be mitigated. He advocates a strong line on obtaining informed consent for research amongst potentially vulnerable groups of patients.

The chapters in this book do not attempt to provide the answers to the difficult and complex moral problems that have been raised and it is not a 'how to do it' book. The purpose of this book is to raise issues and explore ways of thinking about such problems. Those readers who wish to extend their own thinking and enhance the ethical dimensions of their own clinical practice will hopefully find this book both stimulating and engaging.

NOTE

1 For further elaboration on the different types of ethical reasoning see Beauchamp and Childress (1994).

REFERENCES

Beauchamp, T. and Childress, J. (1994) *Principles of Biomedical Ethics*, Oxford: Oxford University Press.

Gillon, R. (1985) *Philosophical Medical Ethics*, Chichester: John Wiley & Sons.

Part I

Themes

Chapter 1

Uncertainty and responsibility

Christopher Dowrick

> [A]t once it struck me what quality went to form a Man of Achievement, especially in Literature, and which Shakespeare possessed so enormously – I mean *Negative Capability*, that is, when a man is capable of being in uncertainties, mysteries, doubts, without any irritable reaching after fact and reason. ...
>
> John Keats (1817)

In this chapter I wish to explore what appears to be a major problem for general practitioners in our work with patients, namely the uncomfortable juxtaposition of uncertainty and responsibility. I shall begin by exploring some of the levels and degrees of uncertainty which exist in ordinary general practice. I shall then describe a set of pragmatic strategies which most of us use to reduce our sense of uncertainty on the one hand, and a second set of strategies which we may use to reduce our sense of responsibility on the other hand. Next I shall discuss the extent to which philosophical concepts drawn from the field of logic – in particular probability theory and decision analysis – can guide our decision making in areas of clinical uncertainty. I shall argue that these can be helpful in specific areas of diagnosis and management. However, they are often limited by our tendency to adopt heuristic ('rule of thumb') biases and, more importantly, they cannot assist us in making decisions in the context of conflicting value systems. In situations of unresolved conflict Levi's 'weighted average principle' may offer us some useful guidance. Finally, I suggest that, far from being an unwanted burden for general practitioners, the tension between uncertainty and responsibility may be an important and necessary motivating force.

LEVELS OF UNCERTAINTY

During a study of doctors and patients on a metabolic research unit in Canada, Renee Fox proposed three basic types of uncertainty affecting physicians: incomplete mastery of available knowledge; limitations in current medical knowledge; and the consequent difficulty of 'distinguishing between personal ignorance or ineptitude and the limitations of present medical knowledge' (Fox, 1959). She also noticed the strategies that the physicians used to cope with the stresses of such uncertainty – 'counter-phobic grim joking', wagering behaviour when predictions were hazardous and devising magical techniques to enable them to carry out their tasks with confidence and poise. Katz (1988) has characterized these behaviours as a *disregard of uncertainty*, an attitude which may result from simple denial, from traditional ideas about the ethical conduct of physicians towards patients or from a sense of the proper exercise of one's professional responsibilities. I think that the uncertainties confronting general practitioners are considerably more complex than this, and our methods of disregarding them consequently tend to be more varied and subtle.

At the same time we (usually) carry with us a sense of a duty to care and do our best for our patients. No matter how patient-centred we may be, how sophisticated our abilities to devolve decision making to or share it with our patients, we believe that it matters what we think and do, that to a greater or lesser degree we do have the power to make things better or worse for patients, even if 'only' to affect how they feel about themselves and their health, and that we must exercise this power in the best possible way.

We are often uncertain about diagnoses. What problems are going to be presented to us by the next patient who comes through the door of the consulting room? We may not be sure whether his fatigue, headache or abdominal pain is the start of a serious and life-threatening condition or will prove to be caused by a straightforward and self-limiting viral infection. It is also often unclear what our patients' perceptions of their problems may be, what ideas they have about how their problems should be managed and what other hidden or complicating psychosocial agendas they may have.

In many cases presented to us there will be room for debate about the best management options. Should we prescribe antibiotics for otitis media or antidepressants for mild to moderate depression? Should we refer patients with prostatic symptoms to a urologist early or indeed at all? There may be a discrepancy between the best and the available management options, for instance in the care of the frail elderly or patients with severe and enduring mental illness. Nor can we be confident that even the best and most comprehensively researched treatment options – such as prescribing aspirin for the secondary prevention of myocardial infarction – will achieve substantial improvement in health of the particular individual patient in front of us.

At more fundamental levels we may be uncertain about the nature of our professional role: are we biomedical scientists, holistic physicians, social workers or health service administrators? We may also be aware that there are conflicting epistemological paradigms – biomedical, psychosocial, political or spiritual, for example – within which we can seek to explain our patients' problems, and that the paradigm within which we operate will affect the type of action we adopt.

The varying levels of uncertainty can be summed up as follows:

Diagnosis	range
	severity
	patient's expectations
	complicating factors
Management	best options
	available options
	efficacy of options
Paradigms	biomedical
	psychosocial
	political
	spiritual, etc.

During the course of a recent routine morning surgery I saw eighteen patients. Eight of them had upper respiratory problems, five were depressed, two each had cardiac and musculoskeletal problems, and there were also requests for my help with impetigo, abdominal pain, contraception and a life insurance form.

After each consultation I made brief notes about any aspects which had caused me uncertainty. In six cases – including abdominal and musculoskeletal pain – my diagnosis was provisional at best. For at least ten of the eighteen patients I was not fully confident about the management options I recommended, ranging from the prescription of antibiotics for an upper respiratory tract infection to a focused psychological intervention for complex marital problems. With six patients I was uncertain about which knowledge paradigm was most appropriate. I found Richard Markham the most troubling of these cases.

Richard is a 59-year-old married man who has worked all his life in a brass foundry. His work is highly specialized and a source of great pride, particularly his contribution to the sculpture of a figure on horseback which is prominently displayed in a city centre churchyard. He came to see me to review ongoing problems with his knees. He reported that the pains in his knees were still there though they had improved since he reduced his working week to three days. I informed him that the X-ray we organized on his last visit has shown no abnormality.

He has two other problems which concerned me. He was extremely anxious, and I suspect probably also depressed. He clearly finds coming to the doctor a very stressful experience and does so as rarely as possible. He is also in a high-risk category for cardiac disease. He had a myocardial infarction when he was 31, has a strong family history of ischaemic heart disease, drinks at least five pints of beer a night and is overweight as well as anxious. Blood tests ordered after his last visit revealed high cholesterol levels and suggested physical damage from his alcohol intake. His blood pressure on this occasion was raised at 180/105. Richard is trying to reduce weight, but is very reluctant to reduce his alcohol intake.

It is clear from a biomedical perspective that in order to reduce his risk of cardiac disease Richard should reduce or stop his consumption of alcohol, and that his musculoskeletal problems will be mitigated if he reduces his hours of work. But a psychosocial approach identifies alcohol as one of his main sources of pleasure and relaxation. And his work has been his main source of personal identity. Which is more important, the quality or the quantity of his life? My uncertainty here is which paradigm to adopt, rather than what advice to give within an assumed biomedical paradigm.

Being uncertain is not a problem if we do not have to act. Having responsibility is not a problem if we know what to do. But if we have to act in a situation when we do not know what to do – that is more difficult. To what extent can ethics help us to address and minimize this difficulty?

PRAGMATIC STRATEGIES TO REDUCE UNCERTAINTY

There are several methods which general practitioners adopt – whether consciously or not – to minimize uncertainty or else to reduce the stress that it may generate. I do not wish to suggest that these methods are intrinsically unethical or wrong, but rather to offer a tentative taxonomy as a basis for critical observation and reflection.

Within consultations general practitioners have a tendency to set limits on the legitimacy of problems presented by patients. We use their initial cues to channel encounters towards a small number of preconceived specific diagnostic and management strategies and interpret any later information received within those terms. We may then ignore 'extraneous' information – particularly relating to psychological and social problems – and fail to respond to or follow patients' verbal agendas (Campion *et al.*, 1992). A study of principals in the former Mersey region found that they were most likely to consider acute physical problems as appropriate or relevant to their knowledge and skills, while social issues were considered least appropriate. It concluded that general practitioners probably work to a *bio(psycho)* rather than a biopsychosocial model of health care (Dowrick *et al.*, 1996).

The majority of general practitioners now work in groups with three or more partners (Fry, 1992). Within such groups there is a tendency for doctors to develop *special interests,* such as asthma, diabetes or mental health. This may happen overtly, after a decision within the practice that one partner should set up a chronic disease clinic. It may also build up by custom and practice over time, with impetus from both partners and patients. A doctor with a particular interest in depression, for example, may receive internal referrals of complicated cases from partners, which will inevitably take up a significant proportion of her time. Receptionists may also steer patients in her direction, and patients themselves will over time tend to gravitate towards her for help with that particular type of problem. The net result is that the likelihood of that doctor seeing a depressed patient during a routine surgery is much higher than usual, thus reducing her level of uncertainty about the range of potential diagnoses and treatment options which she needs to consider.

Financial considerations may also be used to reduce uncertainties in clinical work. It is perfectly legitimate – although ethically dubious – for general practitioners to concentrate their interests and efforts on those aspects of their clinical work which generate the most income. The 1990 GP Contract, for example, has encouraged some doctors to maximize their list sizes in deprived areas, and focus their attention on achieving the highest targets for immunization and cervical cytology and other fee-for-service programmes (Dowrick *et al.*, 1995). The debate within British general practice over core and non-core functions (RCGP, 1996) is also germane to this issue. By specifying the types of problem general practitioners should treat as part of general medical services, and itemizing other tasks for which extra payments should be negotiated, the profession is overtly setting limits on the uncertainty within which it is prepared to operate.

To summarize, a *taxonomy of pragmatic strategies to reduce uncertainty* could be as follows:

In the consultation	select patient cues for response
	bio(psycho) model
In the practice	develop specializations
In the profession	financial orientation
	core and non-core services

PRAGMATIC STRATEGIES TO REDUCE UNCERTAINTY

It is of course possible for general practitioners to alter the other side of the equation by reducing the level of responsibility we assume for the problems presented to us by our patients. Referral behaviours, patient centredness and our professional culture can all be used in this way. As with the taxonomy of strategies to reduce uncertainty, my argument is not that these are unethical per se, but that they can be used to abdicate responsibilities which arguably we should retain.

If we are not sure about diagnosis or management we can *refer*. In the past the most common route of referral was 'upwards' to hospital consultants, providing a major means of shifting responsibility for problems that we found complicated or difficult to manage. Although the overall proportion of cases referred in this direction has remained relatively constant at about 10 per cent (Fry, 1992), there has been a change in the threshold for referral. The increasing sophistication of investigative options available to general practitioners and the pressure to shift care and resources from secondary to primary care mean that we tend to work up cases more comprehensively than in the past before involving our specialist colleagues, and therefore retain more responsibility for diagnosis and management.

However, the expansion of primary health care teams has provided many more opportunities for us to refer 'sideways', to district nurses, physiotherapists or counsellors, for example. While this has many major advantages for effective patient care, there are also potential ethical hazards. Access to these colleagues is usually much more rapid than to a hospital outpatient clinic. They are also likely – either through their terms of employment or a sense of professional subordination – to be amenable to our direct control and influence. We may therefore at times be tempted to ask them to shoulder an excessive burden of responsibility for both diagnosis and management of patients, in a context where it is difficult for them to refuse to do so.

As general practitioners we place great emphasis on the importance of being *patient centred*, of listening carefully to our patients' concerns, their views about the nature of their problems and their opinions about the best methods of managing them (Byrne and Long, 1975). Ethically this concept appears impeccable. It embodies respect for the individual, patient empowerment and a commitment to developing the patient's sense of her ability to manage her own health and disease.

Patient-centredness can, however, merge imperceptibly into a withdrawal of responsibility, a refusal by the doctor to apply himself to an adequate degree of thought and decision making. An extreme but uncomfortably widespread example is the telephone encounter between patient and receptionist in which the patient announces he has tonsillitis and needs an antibiotic and the doctor simply writes a prescription for penicillin to be picked up later. Another common scenario involves the patient with non-specific urethritis, who you are certain has unresolved psychosexual problems, but who simply wants another prescription for trimethoprim. It is so much easier, on a busy Friday evening when you are running thirty minutes late, to reach for the prescription pad than to attempt the complex task of symptom reattribution which will be difficult and distressing for both you and your patient. In the case of my patient Richard Markham it would have been easy for me to limit our consultation to a review of the state of his knees which is the main (indeed probably the only) medical topic which he wished to discuss with me. Patient-centredness can thus be used to avoid the need to enter into genuine dialogue and debate with patients, and become a 'meeting between experts' gone awry. It may also be perceived by our patients as evidence that we do not care about them or indeed as negligent incompetence.[1]

I believe that there must ultimately be some limits on the extent of our willingness to abdicate our responsibility in favour of patient self-determination. John Stuart Mill, in his essay 'On Liberty', proposes a very extensive degree of individual autonomy, but sets limits on the rights of individuals to take actions prejudicial to others and accepts that authorities (governments in his case, doctors in ours) have both rights and obligations to interfere to help individuals (Mill, 1962). An example is the man unknowingly about to drive his coach and horses across a broken bridge. In this case he believes we have a duty to intervene to prevent a dangerous or fatal accident. At some point the professional or personal responsibility of even the most laissez-faire general practitioner will reassert itself, when faced perhaps with a pre-eclamptic woman insisting on a home delivery, an actively suicidal patient, a young man requesting a prescription for substances of abuse or direct evidence of marital violence or child abuse. It may be through consideration of such extreme cases that we can begin to define our personal responses to the ethical boundaries of responsibility between doctors and our patients.

We can use considerations derived from our *professional culture* to avoid or reduce the extent of our personal responsibility for decisions and actions with patients. This may involve undue reliance on the opinions and practices of our trainers or partners, with the possibility of collusion in management options that we ourselves consider to be outdated or incorrect (Griffiths and Luker, 1997).

We may also choose to practice defensive medicine, in the sense that our primary emphasis is on minimizing the risk of complaint or litigation rather than on acting in the best interest of our patients' health. This may lead us, for example, to subject our elderly patients to painful or distressing investigations just to be absolutely sure that we are not missing a carcinoma or, in the case of acute psychiatric conditions, to opt for an early compulsory admission – leading to massively increased personal stress and later socio-economic stigma for the patient – rather than take any degree of risk that the patient may commit suicide.

A *taxonomy of pragmatic strategies to reduce responsibility* can be seen below:

Referral	'upwards'
	'sideways'
Patient-centredness	
Professional culture	trainers and partners
	medico-legal

LOGICAL DECISION MAKING

Responsibility involves both the need and the ability to make decisions, to exercise choices on behalf of other people. There are conceptual tools deriving from logic via statistical theory which offer general practitioners the ability to reduce their degree of uncertainty about clinical problems and hence make decision making easier. This is a major area of fruitful academic activity (see, for example, Dowie and Elstein, 1988), of which I shall briefly describe two strands, probability theory and decision analysis.

Probability theory is a useful way of reducing levels of uncertainty in many clinical situations, particularly in relation to diagnosis. Bayes' theorem governs the way in which our belief in hypotheses should be updated in the light of new information (Phillips, 1973). It can be used as a basis for calculating the probability of an explanation being true, given that the fact is true, from two other sets of information:

1 The probability of those explanations before the fact was known. In the case of medical diagnoses, the probabilities indicate how common are the different illnesses that can give rise to a given symptom. These are often referred to as the *prior odds* of the hypotheses or the *base rates* of the illness. For instance, probabilities can be constructed for the prior odds that a pain in the right iliac fossa is due to an inflamed appendix or that rectal bleeding is caused by a colonic carcinoma.
2 For each hypothesis, the probability of the fact being true given that the hypothesis is true. For diagnoses, these probabilities indicate how likely a particular symptom is given that the patient definitely has the disease and are often referred to as *conditional probabilities*. If a patient has adult onset diabetes, for example, the probability that he will develop retinal or cardiac complications can be estimated.

Decision analysis may be useful in clinical situations where it is not possible to rely on the results of a research trial or to have access to a large database of relevant material (Doubilet and McNeil, 1985), and may be especially helpful as a guide to management. It involves three basic steps:

1 construct a decision tree which displays the available decision options and the possible consequences of each;
2 assign probabilities to uncertain events;
3 assign values or utilities to each possible outcome.

The strategy with the highest expected utility is considered to be the best one. However, the probabilities and values assigned in steps 2 and 3 are unlikely to be fixed or agreed upon by all concerned. It is therefore usual to carry out a fourth step of *sensitivity analysis*, in which the initial assumptions about probabilities and values are systematically altered to determine how sensitive the optimal strategy is to their variation within a reasonable range.

Later in this book Colin Bradley (see Chapter 7) discusses the possible use of decision analysis in general practice prescribing. It could also be helpful in deciding, for example, how to manage a patient with a frozen shoulder. The initial decision tree would include the common general practice options of doing nothing, offering advice and analgesia, offering a local steroid injection, referral to a physiotherapist or referral to an orthopaedic surgeon. If, for the sake of simplicity, we just take the two options of steroid injection (A) or physiotherapy (B), then the possible consequences of each can be predicted. For A they would include anticipatory stress, no benefit, temporary relief of symptoms, permanent relief of symptoms. For B they are similar, though the levels of anticipatory stress are likely to be much lower.

The probabilities and value of each possible outcome for each option will be difficult to determine, and will need a sensitivity analysis involving several versions. For example, the likelihood of steroid injection leading to anticipatory stress might be considered to range from 0.4 to 0.8, and the negative value of this might be taken to range from 0.3 to 0.7. The probability of temporary cure might range from 0.3 to 0.5, and of permanent cure from 0.1 to 0.4. With physiotherapy the cure probabilities would be set lower (say 0.2 to 0.4 for temporary and 0.0 to 0.3 for permanent cures), but so would the outcome of anticipatory stress (say 0.0 to 0.2). In this example the balance in favour of option A or option B would be significantly affected by the size of the probability and negative value placed on anticipatory stress.

The *decision tree for managing a frozen shoulder* can be set out as follows:

OPTION	OUTCOME	PROBABILITY	VALUE
Steroid injection	anticipatory stress	0.4 to 0.8	–0.3 to –0.7
	no benefit	0.2 to 0.5	0
	temporary benefit	0.3 to 0.5	0.7 to 0.9
	permanent benefit	0.1 to 0.4	1
Physiotherapy	anticipatory stress	0.0 to 0.2	–0.3 to –0.7
	no benefit	0.3 to 0.6	0
	temporary benefit	0.2 to 0.4	0.7 to 0.9
	permanent benefit	0.0 to 0.2	1

Probability theory and decision analysis are valuable tools for reducing uncertainty and making it easier for general practitioners to exercise their responsibilities rationally. However, their usefulness has both theoretical and practical limitations.[2] When human beings make probabilistic judgements about everyday situations we do not consider the available options in a purely rational manner, but often make gross errors. Kahneman *et al.* (1982) have described how we tend to use *heuristic* ('rule of thumb') methods for assessing probabilities. They divide these methods into three broad categories:

1 *Representativeness*. A person, thing or event is judged to be a member of a class whose stereotypical members it closely resembles, regardless of other information such as the relative size of those classes. For example, if members of a group of students are asked to decide whether Linda is more likely to be a bank teller, or a bank teller who is active in the feminist movement, they will tend to select the second option. They do so because it more closely approximates to their own choices, and disregard the simple logic that feminist bank tellers must by definition be a subset of all bank tellers. Similarly, if general practitioners are asked whether Sharon is more likely to be a lone parent, or a lone parent who is depressed, we may tend to choose the second option because it more closely represents our views of what lone parents are like.

2 *Availability*. Probability may be judged by the ease with which instances can be brought to mind, by their availability from memory. Therefore we tend to overestimate the frequency of highly publicized but comparatively rare events such as air crashes. In medical terms this may lead us to overestimate the frequency of diseases which have a high public profile, such as AIDS or Creutzfeld-Jacob Disease. We may also overestimate the frequency of conditions which have a high personal profile. For instance, if we have recently 'missed' a case of childhood meningitis we are likely to make this diagnosis for a much higher proportion of febrile headaches after the event than we did previously, even though the actual prevalence or likelihood will not have altered at all.

3 *Anchoring and adjustment*. This heuristic device involves taking an initial value or anchor, and then adjusting it. The anchor may be suggested by the formulation of the problem or it may be the result of a partial computation. For example, a general practitioner may be used – by following the examples of her colleagues or because she is concerned about dangers of side effects – to treating depressive disorders with 25mg of amitriptyline daily. If she reads an article advocating higher dosages of antidepressant medication she will start from the anchor of 25mg and adjust her dosages in steps commensurate with this. She is therefore much more likely to increase her standard prescribing to 50mg of amitriptyline rather than the currently recommended 150mg daily dosage.

Probability theory and decision analysis are of limited help when faced with uncertainty over competing value judgements. I am here taking a Kantian rather than a Cartesian perspective and assuming that value judgements are in the realm of metaphysics and as such must ultimately be accepted as *a priori* positions beyond the reach of logic. They may be informed by and expanded through logic, but are intrinsically irrefutable by it (Kant, 1996). In general philosophical terms Christianity, Marxism and psychoanalysis are examples of metaphysics, of paradigms which can be explored by but not explained by logic (Dowrick, 1983).[3] In general practice terms, so are the dilemmas posed by my patient Richard Markham, whose problems troubled me because I could formulate them in either biomedical or psychosocial terms yet was unable to find a way of deciding which of these value systems or paradigms was the more important. In the final section of this chapter I turn to the American philosopher Isaac Levi for help with this difficulty.

DECISION MAKING UNDER UNRESOLVED CONFLICT

If we find ourselves in a position where there is a conflict of value systems, and in which there is no obvious reason why one should take priority over the other, Levi argues that we should avoid coming to a conclusion as to what ought categorically to be done when, all things considered, no verdict is warranted or possible. Instead we should aim to adopt a position which is as acceptable as possible within each value system.

> if the agent starts committed to two or more value systems which on the occasion mandate different rankings of the feasible options, he should avoid contradiction by moving to a position of suspense which avoids prejudicing the resolution of the conflict among rival value commitments.
>
> (Levi, 1986: 10)

Levi proposes the technical concept of *the weighted average principle* as a method of resolving such conflicts.

> Assume V(U) = value structure V for determining permissible ways of evaluating feasible options in set U. If $v_1, v_2, \ldots v_n$ (*n* finite) are *v*-functions permissible in V(U) which are not positive affine transformations of one another (and, hence, represent distinct ways of evaluation), then for every n-tuple $<w_1, w_2, \ldots, w_n>$ of nonnegative weights which sum to 1, the weighted average $\Sigma\, w_i v_i$ is also permissible.
>
> (Levi, 1986: 78)

When there are two or more permissible rankings, the set of options optimal according to one need not coincide with the set of options optimal to another.

A simple example would be of a general practitioner seeking to employ a practice manager who is skilled both in managing reception staff and in negotiating fundholding budgets with the local health authority. Three people apply for the vacancy: A is an excellent people manager, but has no experience of financial matters; B was a finance officer in a local business, but has no experience of personnel; C is reasonably competent at both tasks, but is less impressive than A at the first or B at the second. If the general practitioner considers good staff relations to be her main concern she should offer the job to A, or if fundholding is the priority she should offer it to B. But if she is equally committed to good staff relations and to maximizing her fundholding opportunities she should choose to employ C because the weighted average of benefit will be greater to the practice than if she employs either A or B.

Levi also accepts a *hierarchy of value structures*: if options are equally admissible at the highest hierarchy, we can move onto a second level value system. This process can be iterated any finite number of times. The general practitioner decides that fundholding is her main priority, and finds that D has also applied for the job. D and B have very similar financial and business acumen, but D is Afro-Caribbean while B is Caucasian. The options at the highest hierarchy are now equally admissible, so she can now consider a second level value system relating in this case to the possibilities for positive discrimination for people from disadvantaged ethnic communities.

How does all this help me decide what advice to offer to Richard Markham? If I accept that biomedical and psychosocial value systems are both permissible, then in evaluating feasible management options I should seek to deploy those options which will lead to maximum potential benefit within both value systems. This may mean discarding certain options which would be considered of higher benefit if only one value system were permissible.

If I take a purely psychosocial paradigm I will encourage Richard to maintain his sense of identity and self-esteem by continuing to work in the brass foundry (though easing off a bit to preserve his knees) and frequenting his local public house as usual. A biomedical focus on reducing risk factors for cardiac disease could lead me to offer forthright advice about the dangers inherent in his levels of alcohol intake and his weight and raises the likelihood of long-term antihypertensive medication. The weighted average principle leads towards a median position in which the problems of alcohol and diet are discussed within the context of a life-style that has many positive aspects, and in which any proposals for antihypertensive medication (and hence for regular stress-inducing contact with the medical profession) are delayed for as long as possible.

The case for exploring and treating Richard's anxiety and possible depression is admissible within either system, and second level value options can therefore be considered. The question of a preference for (equally effective) psychological or pharmacological approaches to the treatment of minor psychiatric conditions could be considered at this level.

The potential for uncertainty in a case like this is probably infinite. There is a further theoretical and practical problem posed by possible differences between Richard's needs (however they may be defined) and his desires. It may be that these also have to be taken as equally permissible value systems, adding yet more complexity to the matrix. Nor can I be sure how influential my advice is actually likely to be, regardless of the excellence and depth of its philosophical pedigree, in affecting what decisions Richard makes about his work and his attitude to health.

AN ETHIC OF UNCERTAINTY

In this chapter I have attempted to address the problem posed by the need for general practitioners to act as responsibly as possible in conditions of considerable uncertainty. I have drawn attention to some of the methods we commonly use to minimize the tensions caused by this dilemma. I have described an alternative set of logical and ethical methods for resolving these tensions, including probability theory, decision analysis and the weighted average principle.

I am aware that there can be no final comfortable answers to the tension between uncertainty and responsibility. Perhaps this is as it should be. In the quotation at the head of this chapter, John Keats – physician as well as poet – reminds us of the wisdom and maturity needed to achieve 'negative capability', to remain in 'uncertainties, mysteries, doubts, without any irritable reaching after fact and reason'.

It may be that we should accept – and welcome – this tension as an ethical or ontological position in its own right. Without it we could too easily become bored, stale and ineffective.

In his beautiful and compelling description of John Sassall, a British country doctor in the 1960s, Berger compares him with Joseph Conrad's Master Mariner, who went to sea to combat the boredom and complacency of middle-class life in England. For the doctor the equivalent of the sea was single-handed general practice in an economically and culturally deprived part of rural England. Berger describes how Sassall's curiosity, his spirit of enquiry, his desire to experience all that is possible, his need to find cases where no previous given explanation would fit, were the essential ingredients which kept his own imagination (and hence himself) alive. 'Sassall needs his unsatisfied quest for certainty and his uneasy sense of unlimited responsibility' (Berger, 1997: 88).

So perhaps do we all. It may be that this conflict, this dilemma, is what motivated many of us to enter general practice in the first place. It may also be the basis on which, despite our frequent protestations to the contrary, our energy and our enthusiasm can flourish.

Key points

- Uncertainty and responsibility are central factors in general practice.
- Uncertainties exist at many levels of practice.
- We adopt pragmatic strategies to reduce our sense of uncertainty and our sense of responsibility.
- Logical decision making techniques can help to reduce uncertainty in diagnosis and management.
- When value systems conflict, decisions should be taken which reflect the 'best fit' with all the relevant value systems.
- The tension between uncertainty and responsibility may be what keeps general practitioners alive and well!

NOTES

1 See also Len Doyal's discussion on genuine and spurious patient autonomy in Chapter 3.
2 See also Lucy Frith's discussion of the limitations of evidence based medicine in Chapter 2.
3 See also Sam Smith's discussion of conflicting views about the status of medical knowledge in Chapter 6.

REFERENCES

Berger, J. (1997) *A Fortunate Man: The Story of a Country Doctor*, New York: Vintage International.

Byrne, P.S. and Long, B.E.L. (1975) *Learning to Care: Person to Person*, Edinburgh: Churchill Livingstone.

Campion, P., Butler, N. and Cox, A. (1992) 'Principal agendas of doctors and patients in general practice consultations', *Family Practice* 9: 181–90.

Doubilet, P. and McNeil, B. (1985) 'Clinical decision making', *Medical Care* 2: 648–62.

Dowie, J. and Elstein, A. (1988) *Professional Judgement: A Reader in Clinical Decision Making*, Cambridge: Cambridge University Press.

Dowrick, C. (1983) 'Strange meeting: Marxism, psychoanalysis and social work', *British Journal of Social Work* 13: 1–18.

Dowrick, C., May, C., Richardson, M. and Bundred, P. (1996) 'The biopsychosocial model of general practice: rhetoric or reality?', *British Journal of General Practice* 46: 105–7.

Dowrick, C., May, C., Richardson, M. and Choudhry, N. (1995) *Evaluation of the North West Regional Health Authority Primary Care Initiative: Report for the Period 1994–5*, Department of Primary Care, University of Liverpool.

Fox, R. (1959) *Experiment Perilous: Physicians and Patients Facing the Unknown*, Glencoe Ill: Free Press.

Fry, J. (1992) *General Practice: The Facts*, Oxford: Radcliffe Medical Press.

Griffiths, J.M. and Luker, K.A. (1997) 'A barrier to clinical effectiveness: the etiquette of district nursing', *Clinical Effectiveness in Nursing* 1(3): 121–8.

Kahneman, D., Slovic, P. and Tversky, A. (eds) (1982) *Judgement under Uncertainty: Heuristics and Biases*, Cambridge: Cambridge University Press.

Kant, I. (1996) *The Metaphysic of Morals*, Cambridge: Cambridge University Press.

Katz, J.(1988) 'Why doctors don't disclose uncertainty', in J. Dowie and A. Elstein (eds) *Professional Judgement: A Reader in Clinical Decision Making*, Cambridge: Cambridge University Press.

Levi, I. (1986) *Hard Choices: Decision Making Under Unresolved Conflict*, Cambridge: Cambridge University Press.

Mill, J.S. (1962) 'On Liberty', in Mary Warnock (ed.) *John Stuart Mill*, London: Collins/Fontana.

Phillips, L.D. (1973) *Bayesian Statistics For Social Scientists*, London: Nelson.

Royal College of General Practitioners (1996) *Report 27: The Nature of General Medical Practice*, London: RCGP.

Chapter 2

Evidence-based medicine and general practice

Lucy Frith

There have been relatively few critical evaluations of evidence-based medicine (EBM).[1] This is partly because of the novelty of the enterprise: it is only since the early 1990s that the term has had general currency, although the closely related outcomes based research has had a longer history in the United States.[2] However, another reason for the lack of critical gaze is that EBM appears to rest on an innocuous truism, a point amusingly made by a modern Socrates questioning Enthusiasticus, a supporter of EBM. 'I thought that all doctors were trained in the scientific tradition, one tenet of which is to examine the evidence on which their practice is based. How then does this new evidence-based medicine differ from traditional medicine?' (Grahame-Smith,1995: 1126). EBM does not differ from traditional medicine because it insists that medical practice should be based on evidence, rather EBM takes a different definition of what is good medical evidence and what are appropriate mechanisms for finding and evaluating this evidence.

The aim of this chapter is not to criticize the central premise of EBM, that medical practice should be based on some form of evidence, nor to question the nature of the evidence nor the mechanisms for finding it. The aim is, rather, to consider how this evidence is employed in practice, how it affects clinical decision making. EBM attempts to make clinical decision making 'better', that is more scientific and less based on individual opinion. Clinical trials produce scientific data on a treatment's effects and this can then be used by clinicians to make more objective treatment decisions. For the purposes of this chapter, I shall accept for the sake of argument that the data trials produce are sound and not subject to errors. I shall argue that the use of EBM involves some form of interpretation of the data, which is essential if the data are to be applied to treatment decisions, and this interpretation is a non-objective process and one that incorporates value judgements. Thus, treatment decisions may be based on objective, scientific data but this does not mean that the decision itself is objective, as the decision will have involved an interpretation and evaluation of the data.

I will first examine what proponents of EBM mean by a better, more objective clinical decision and then I shall show how interpretation and evaluation of the data are essential for applying the data in practice. Finally, I will examine the use of EBM in practice, its application in general practice and the use of best evidence clinical guidelines.

EBM AND OBJECTIVITY

The aim of EBM is to ground medical practice on good evidence so that the treatments patients receive are both the most effective and the least harmful. Therefore, patients, so it is claimed, will get the 'best' medical treatment based on the current state of knowledge. 'It is the objective nature by which the EBM paradigm approaches the question of "what are we doing" and "how can we do better" that causes health care providers and funding agencies to increasingly adopt this paradigm as a primary principle' (Cooper *et al.*, 1996: 778).

EBM has gained popularity due to a perceived improvement in the standard of medical evidence. It is this improvement in medical evidence that is a crucial factor in the claim that clinical decisions can be made more objectively. Davidoff *et al.* argue that, 'what has changed in clinical medicine in recent decades is the very nature of clinical evidence itself.' (1995a: 727). According to Davidoff *et al.*,[3] the quality of medical evidence is improving by becoming more objective and therefore more reliable. They highlight three changes in clinical evidence. First, the standards for gathering information have altered. Previously, the standard unit of clinical information was an individual patient, represented in the case report. However, this older anecdotal form of evidence has been replaced by a new epidemiological standard, which has raised the standard for the acceptable level of etiologic and diagnostic evidence. 'Case reports have yielded to population-derived studies of which the randomized control trial is the prototype or "gold-standard" of therapeutic evidence' (*Ibid.*). By 'raising the standard of evidence' the authors mean that evidence is now more objective and less likely to include subjective error.

Second, the means for assessing and interpreting clinical evidence was formerly basic biostatistics; now this has been expanded to include sophisticated concepts and techniques of experimental trial design, decision analysis and clinical epidemiology. A further change is the belief that 'the concept that a single study, although it might provide the truth, is often not enough. The whole truth may require a synthesis of the evidence from all the best studies, optimally through the use of meta-analysis' (*Ibid.*).

Third, in the past, expert opinion carried as much weight as clinical scientific record. Although Davidoff *et al.* recognize that medicine is still an authoritarian discipline, doctors are encouraged to base their decisions on evidence rather than on the authoritarian utterances of senior colleagues. 'Authoritarian medicine may thus be gradually yielding to authoritative medicine' (*Ibid.*). In summary of Davidoff *et al.*'s points, the main change in clinical evidence is the reliance on the results of randomized control trials (RCT) or other robust experimental studies. In order for evidence to be characterized as 'good' the evidence should be produced by clinical trials and ideally a randomized control trial.

Due to this improvement there has been an increasing concern to implement this good evidence in clinical practice. This is a concern expressed by many commentators, for example Davidoff *et al.* argue that 'there is a widening chasm between what we ought to do and what we actually do' (1995a: 1085). Such a delay in employing research evidence in clinical practice has arguably resulted in expensive, ineffectual or even harmful decision making. EBM aims to employ the results of clinical trials in medical practice, thus bridging the gap between research and practice.

An important element in this improvement of medical evidence is the use of systematic reviews. Systematic reviews are designed to make clinical decision making more objective. The reviews are a formal process to eliminate what could be termed clinical judgement, to replace a subjective process with an objective one for appraising clinical evidence. The use of systematic reviews is designed to replace the clinician's individual assessment of the data with a clearly defined, impartial and hence objective, process.

With the advent of this improvement of medical evidence the individual experiences of the doctor are now viewed to be an inadequate grounding for decision making. This type of decision making has been categorized as containing some or all of the following elements: a reliance on case studies, anecdotal cases of previous patients and the personal dissemination of clinical experience where individual expertise is as important as research findings.[4] These deliberations combine information gathered from laboratory science (the anatomical and physiological aspects of organisms) and subjective elements that comprise personal knowledge and the assessment of the individual patient. In this way doctors are seen to be basing their clinical decisions on opinion derived from their own experience; this type of knowledge is derided because it is not solely based on firm evidence and hence not objectively verifiable. Tanenbaum sums up this approach by saying clinical decision making is 'more like deliberation than calculation, insightful as well as informed, a gestalt or story rather than algorithm' (1995: 1270).

Such a view of medical decision making is problematic for supporters of EBM as it is too reliant on the skills and qualities of the individual doctor. By employing an explicit process of decision making, that of a systematic review, it is claimed that the subjective judgement of the doctor can be removed and therefore decisions made more objectively. This process begins by the doctor conducting a systematic review of the research evidence and then combining the results of the primary studies to produce what is termed a meta-analysis of the results.

> Meta-analysis is a quantitative approach for systematically combining the results of previous research in order to arrive at conclusions about the body of research. Studies of a topic are systematically identified. Criteria for including and excluding studies are defined, and data from eligible studies are abstracted. Last, the data are combined statistically, yielding a quantitative estimate of the size of the effect of treatment and a test of homogeneity in the estimate of effect size.
>
> (Petitti, 1994: 5)

Mulrow (1995) comments that, although sometimes arduous and time consuming, this methodology is usually quicker and less costly than embarking on a new study. This methodology can also be supported by the argument that it is more ethical to gather information from studies already done than conduct new ones and subject further patients to the potential risks and harms of a RCT.

The most important aspect of meta-analysis is the criteria that delineate an acceptable study for inclusion in the review. The main criterion for the inclusion of a study in a systematic review is that it is a randomized controlled study. Although meta-analyses admit the use of other types of studies, these are often only recommended if no suitable randomized studies have been conducted. Once the relevant studies have been found they must be evaluated against a predetermined checklist to ensure two main aims. First, that the studies have produced a significant result. For example, what was the size of the treatment effect; how precise was the treatment effect and do the conclusions flow from the evidence that is reviewed? Second, that the study was methodologically sound. For example, were the procedures of randomization adequate and were the researchers blinded to the treatment protocols? If there are defined criteria then this 'explicitness about how decisions were made enables others to assess how well the process protected against errors' (Oxman,1995: 76). Sackett *et al.* (1991), for example, argue that the important aspect of EBM is to make explicit non-explicit clinical reasoning. Hence, the focus of attention is on the methodology of the decision process and there is a belief that once this process is followed a 'better' decision will be made.

These claims, that clinical decisions can be made more objectively by using EBM, are based on two underlying assumptions. First, that there is rigorous evidence available on which to base treatment decisions. It is presupposed that this evidence is objective in the ontological sense, that is to say it exists independently of any perceptions people may have of it and hence is a more accurate picture of reality. Second, that by a clearly defined scientific process that is non-subjective and not open to individual interpretation it is possible to gain access to this objective evidence and hence use this evidence to make an objective clinical decision. It is claimed that EBM, by the use of systematic reviews, provides such a process.

These assumptions are based on a realist view of the world which is broadly the belief that reality exists independently of us and our perceptions of it and that if we employ the right methods we can have knowledge of this reality. Papineau states that realism involves the conjunction of two theses: '(1) *an independence thesis*: our judgements answer for their truth to a world which exists independently of our awareness of it; (2) *a knowledge thesis*: by and large, we can know which of these judgements are true' (1996: 2). It is from this realist assumption that EBM gathers much of its force. This type of evidence is stripped of personal opinion and value judgement and reveals what actually *is* the case. Thus, it is claimed, that we can know for sure what are effective treatments.

The first assumption that there is rigorous evidence available and that this evidence is an improvement on previous forms of medical evidence will be accepted. However, I will argue that proponents of EBM confuse the existence of this more objective evidence with the claim that it is possible to make objective treatment decisions. I will argue that the interpretation of the evidence produced by clinical trials, which is essential if it is to be applied to treatment decisions, is a non-objective process and one that incorporates value judgements. Further, despite the process of systematic review which is seen to improve the objectivity of decision making, there is still an important and unavoidable role for the individual interpretation of the evidence by the clinician when it is applied in practice.

CRITICISMS OF EBM

I will now consider the argument that to apply clinical trial results involves some form of interpretation that incorporates non-objective value-judgements, namely a judgement of what is to be called a good outcome. It is generally argued that clinical trials are designed to find out certain effects of a drug, for example the lowering of plasma cholesterol levels, these effects are capable of being measured by a piece of laboratory equipment. The findings that this equipment produces will be independent of the experimenters' perceptions and hence can be said to objective. This point will be accepted. However, I will argue that the significance given to the effect and whether that effect is to be termed a good outcome are not factors inherent in the data but the values we ourselves impose on the data.

RCTs are designed to produce data on the effectiveness of a treatment. These trials can be organized in two ways. First, by comparing the new treatment with a placebo and second by comparing it with an existing treatment. The clinical trial, that seeks to provide information on the comparison between a new treatment and/or a placebo and an existing treatment, is a practical technique to enable clinicians to make working comparisons between different treatments. These trials are often called intention-to-treat trials as they are designed to establish the clinical effect of the drug or treatment. The purpose of intention-to-treat trials is to assess whether a drug works not how it works. They provide information on what treatment is *better* than another or more *effective* than a placebo. It is in this assessment of what makes a treatment better than another that trials incorporate evaluative elements. The researcher makes a value judgement as to whether a particular effect is good or bad and hence whether the treatment is effective. Effectiveness, good outcomes, a 'better' treatment are not pre-existing facts waiting to be discovered by medical science: they are value-laden assessments of the weight given to a particular effect of the treatment. Thus, to say a treatment is effective is summing up one's opinion on the data.

For example, a clinical trial may produce data that say that treatment *x* has a 48 per cent success rate in treating a given condition. Such data do not automatically tell us whether this treatment is an effective treatment for our given condition and whether we should recommend it to our patients. Our assessment of how good the 48 per cent success rate is cannot be objectively determined, but is dependent on a number of factors. First, the severity of the condition being treated. If a condition is life threatening a 48 per cent chance of success would be very good and the treatment would be judged to be very effective. Second, the acceptable level of side-effects of this treatment will depend on the type of condition that is treated. If the condition is life threatening we will bear very bad side-effects to achieve this 48 per cent success rate (for example, the side-effects of chemotherapy are very severe but held to be acceptable). However, for a minor complaint we would not see such side-effects as acceptable and not class the treatment as an effective one. Third, the existence of other treatments and how the new treatment compares will influence how effective we judge our treatment to be. Here cost could also be a delineating factor if two treatments have the same effectiveness but one is cheaper than the other. If there is another treatment *y* with a 60 per cent success rate and comparable side-effects, our treatment will not be seen as effective. If treatment *y* has much worse side-effects than our treatment *x*, determining which treatment is most effective will be a matter of individual clinical judgement and will depend on the preferences of the patient who will receive the treatment.

Brazier cites an example that illustrates this point:

> A woman is told that radical mastectomy will maximise her prospects of recovery from breast cancer. She knows that if she loses a breast her husband will leave her and she knows that psychologically she is unable to cope with the necessary mutilation.
>
> (Brazier, 1992: 88)

Hence she opts for the marginally less 'safe' option of lumpectomy. She is concerned both with the success rate and the consequences for her life and relationships - the side-effects. Here this woman's assessment of which treatment is most effective could be different from another patient's assessment. A different woman may choose a mastectomy as she is less concerned about losing a breast and wants the treatment that has a slightly higher success rate. This illustrates that effectiveness is a relative concept, relative to the individual who receives the treatment.

An argument against this position is that it could be said that it is not important that the results produced by clinical trials incorporate a particular view of what defines a good outcome. If we can formulate a general consensus over what constitutes a good outcome then this can provide an adequate foundation for non-subjective agreement over outcomes. I would respond to this argument by raising two points. In the first place, it is very hard to gain consensus over what constitutes a good outcome. Even basic imperatives like preserving life can be contentious in certain situations. For instance patients in persistent vegetative states, if correctly diagnosed, will never recover from the coma and it has been argued that simply preserving their life is unwarranted. Second, even if a consensus can be reached it is still important to recognize that this is a particular view of a good outcome and it is possible that in different times (or places) a different view of a good outcome could prevail.

In conclusion, if it is accepted that clinical trials produce generally accepted factual data about the interaction of particular drugs or therapies, how can these facts establish which course of action should follow from them? 'The evidence itself will not automatically dictate patient care but will provide the factual basis on which decisions can be made' (Rosenberg and Donald,1995: 1124). No matter how good one's evidence is, it will not automatically determine which course of treatment should be recommended. This is explicitly recognized in articles explaining how to carry out systematic reviews. Once the systematic review has been performed, the clinician 'must decide how (if at all) this numerical result, whether significant or not, should influence the care of an individual patient' (Greenhalgh,1997: 674). The external validity and relevance of the trial has to be assessed by the clinician in relation to the patient. The clinician's evaluation of the empirical data and the application of the evidence to the individual patient is a step that is often obscured, but not removed, in EBM. A systematic review produces information on which to base a clinical decision; it is not the clinical decision itself.

For example, a patient comes to see his GP for a routine check up and it is found that the patient's blood pressure is very high. The GP has a large amount of research evidence that tells her that certain drugs will have the effect of lowering blood pressure. She has no reason to doubt this evidence as a drug that lowers blood pressure can have easily measurable effects. In this case there is good evidence from research trials to indicate what treatment will lower blood pressure. However, the fact that a certain drug will lower blood pressure does not automatically indicate what management strategy should be adopted. There are side-effects and risks of such treatments to take into account, some patients do not like to take medication, others would be better off with changing lifestyle habits. It also presupposes some view of what hypertension is. Is it a disease that needs treating or a risk factor that needs modification? Further, there are the complexities of recommending the treatment in practice as by highlighting raised blood pressure as a condition needing treatment the patient is labelled as 'ill' and this can have consequences for the patient's emotional state. Patients' views and expectations are all vital factors in the success or failure of a treatment, if only on the level of ensuring compliance. Hence, when deciding what management strategies to adopt for hypertension, information from systematic reviews will only provide one piece of the jigsaw.

EBM claims that by using evidence that is of a higher quality, more scientific and more objective, it can make clinical decision making more objective. This is, to my mind, a confusion between two different things, the quality of evidence and the decision. While a decision that is made on the basis of good evidence will be of a higher quality, it will not be more objective in the sense that it is independent of value judgements or our perceptions and priorities. The evidence may be more objective, but the decision is not as it necessarily incorporates the values of those making the decision. This confusion leads to the belief that the evidence will indicate the course of action to be taken and that it is possible to locate the *best* treatment for a condition. I shall consider the practical implications of this belief in the next section.

THE PRACTICAL IMPLEMENTATION OF EBM

I shall now focus on how EBM is used in clinical decision making. With the belief that it is possible to locate one best treatment or a range of specific treatments, it has been suggested that clinical guidelines should be used that are formulated on the basis of the 'best' evidence. Clinical guidelines are an attempt to introduce evidence-based practice at an institutional level, to ensure that medical care is evidence based and everyone receives the best treatment. As argued above, even by using the process of EBM the data still has to be interpreted and an evaluation of how applicable the data is to the individual patient still needs to take place. Whereas, clinical guidelines trade on the belief that it is possible to establish what are the best treatments across the board. The concern here is that clinical guidelines might preclude an assessment of the suitability of a treatment for a particular individual.

A way of incorporating EBM in practice at an institutional, not an individual, level is by the formulation of evidence-based clinical guidelines. The formulation of protocols and guidelines removes the need for individual doctors to have to process the information for themselves by conducting their own systematic review. The NHS Executive has stated, 'on the advice of the Clinical Outcomes Group, [they have] begun to commend a selected number of high quality guidelines' (1996: 20). These guidelines are to be used to inform the clinical management of various groups of illness. Protocols will be formulated by national experts in the field, who will be up to date and informed about the most recent research data[5] and will have conducted the relevant systematic reviews of the literature. These guidelines are an attempt to provide a consistent package of care throughout the NHS, rather than allowing treatments to vary depending on the area in which they are given. The rationale behind these guidelines is that of treating similar cases in the same way, because unwarranted variation in managing similar cases is seen as a core problem for health care providers (James,1993).

However, treatments which produce the desired effect can differ from person to person. Even patients with identical manifestations of a particular disease could give a different weight to various outcomes depending on personal taste, social and family situations, life priorities and so on.[6] The introduction of guidelines might preclude an individual assessment of what is best for that particular patient.

However, supporters of clinical guidelines might argue against this view of the treatment process. They could argue that there are enough similarities between patients suffering from the same condition to see them as being members of the same patient group (in statistical language forming part of the same reference class of patient). Therefore, all that needs to be established is which group the patient belongs to and then the appropriate clinical guideline can be followed. Patrick Suppes, for example, has argued that a decision regarding the individual patient can be extrapolated from other cases. Even though patients may vary in many respects (age, wealth, etc.), 'the direct medical consequences and the direct financial cost of a given method of treatment are the most important consequences, and these can be evaluated by summing across the patients and ignoring more individual features' (1979: 151). Suppes is right in one respect. It may be possible to construct broad generalizations about patients' preferences for certain medical consequences. However, these would have to remain at a very broad level as many of the individual factors affecting these consequences are ignored. For example, financial cost may not be an issue for someone very wealthy, whereas for others even the cost of a simple prescription could be prohibitive. Others may value their life only in so far as they are able to look after their children. Although it might be possible to ascertain the types of consequences that are, on the whole, most important, it is impossible to predetermine their respective value objectively.

It can also be questioned if all medical activity can have specified outcomes and a determined process that can be enshrined in a guideline. Chronic diseases and the effects of ageing, a substantial part of general practice case loads, are not areas in which outcome measurements can be precisely quantified. Hopkins and Solomon make this point, arguing that while guidelines may be useful for surgical procedures or acute illnesses, the care of the elderly and the chronically ill is largely based on support, reassurance and explanation,

> for which the technical interventions available do not influence outcome very much. ... The implicit contract here is not based on process and outcome measures but on mutual trust between doctors and patients that the doctors will provide the best care they can within budgetary constraints.
>
> (1996: 476)

Hopkins and Solomon illustrate this point with the example of the management of stroke patients. They say that the course of the treatment and the outcomes of rehabilitation cannot be predetermined because each person's disability is unique. Hence the therapist has to concentrate on the goals and needs of the particular patient.

Guidelines rely on patient homogeneity, that is patients being very similar. In stroke rehabilitation, where patient variation is high, it is difficult to write a precisely defined clinical guideline. There are on the other hand areas of health care where patient variation is much lower, the removal of wisdom teeth, for example. When this is the case guidelines can be useful. 'In conditions such as day case surgery, a single patient record is easy to introduce. In an intensive care setting, where variations are more common, a pathway together with freehand documentation may be more suitable' (Kitchiner and Bundred, 1996: 166). There are areas where guidelines are more applicable. However, this should not be extended to areas of health care provision where guidelines may be inappropriate. Even when patients are suffering from the same condition guidelines should not be applied unthinkingly. Room should be made for the needs and wants of the patient to be accommodated.

It could be claimed that general practice is an unsuitable area for the widespread introduction of guidelines because GPs are concerned as much with patients' situations and lifestyles as organic medical matters. Hence, due to the individual nature of many treatment decisions, it could be difficult to produce guidelines that reflect each patient's treatment preferences and social situation. A guideline may produce good clinical outcomes for the majority or a substantial majority of patients. However, some patients may not receive the care they want or care that is appropriate for them.

An example of the needs of one patient not being met by the strict application of a clinical guideline is the case cited by Tingle (1996),

Wickline v *State of California 1986*. The California Medicade programme (Medi-Cal) refused a doctor's request for additional days of patient monitoring on the grounds that they were not required under the clinical algorithms developed by Medi-Cal. The patient was discharged and developed complications. She sued Medi-Cal for negligence, arguing that she had been discharged solely on the grounds of cost. The court ruled in her favour, saying physicians should not disregard good medical judgement for cost reasons. Thus it has been argued that 'care paths must be scientifically based and never distorted solely to effect cost control or other non-scientific support' (Segar, quoted in Tingle, 1996). As Tingle states,

> Patient and health carer choice are factors which clearly impact on the *appropriateness* of the application of the clinical guideline. Some clinical guidelines in the USA have written warnings on the front of them stating that they must not be automatically applied and that the clinical judgement of the health carer must always be exercised first. (1997: 640)

This raises the complex issue of the relationship between cost-effectiveness and effectiveness of treatment. In a NHS Executive document on promoting clinical effectiveness by the implementation of guidelines, it states that the aim is 'to ensure that decisions about the provision and delivery of NHS services are increasingly driven by the evidence of clinical and cost-effectiveness ... to ensure the greatest gain from available resources' (NHS Executive, 1996: 6). Here cost is highlighted as a constraining factor and one that will delineate the context of health gain.

In sum, clinical guidelines could restrict a patient's ability to receive the treatment that is most suitable for them. One possible way of protecting the welfare of the individual is to ensure that the patient always gives informed consent to any procedure. It is ethically desirable to get informed consent as a way both of respecting the autonomy and safeguarding the best interests of the individual. To allow patients to make their own decisions about their health care – to respect autonomy – is one of the fundamental ethical requirements of medical practice. Consent is also one of the best ways of ensuring that the medical care given is in the best interests of the patient, as it is thought that the individual concerned will be the best person to promote his/her own interests.

However, with the implementation of guidelines the patient is only offered a choice within a limited range of options. If the treatment that would most benefit the individual is not offered then consent in this context becomes a negative action, in that the act of consent can only be to refuse an option that might be inappropriate. It is not to positively choose an option which may be most beneficial to the patient. Such a refusal clearly does little to safeguard a patient's interests because it does not provide the desired treatment. For instance, a woman might want to have a home birth but finds that in her area there is not the community midwifery support to enable her to do this and her GP will not support her. She opts for a hospital birth, but one that allows her to go home a few hours after the delivery. It can be said that she consents to this hospital birth *and* has not received the kind of care she wanted.

Regarding these points, it could be countered that patients inevitably face a restricted range of the options in any large health care system. The general practitioner cannot refer the patient for a treatment if it is not offered by a local hospital trust. Therefore, when deciding what treatment is appropriate both patient and doctor are constrained by the available options. However, the worry with the introduction of guidelines is that the limited flexibility that currently exists may be reduced even further. This is because the rationale behind guidelines is to recommend the best treatment. This is based on the belief that it is possible to locate the best treatment by using the results of research trials that determine this objectively. Rather the best treatment could be seen as a relative concept; relative to the individual patient.

As informed consent does nothing to safeguard a patient's interests, some other ethical safeguard is needed. Rather than the interests of the wider community of patients becoming paramount, the doctor's therapeutic obligation to the individual patient must remain an important feature of modern medical practice. Greenberg (1994) argues that the increasing focus on the doctor as a health care provider rather than as a clinician leads to the doctor becoming more concerned with the general provision of health care than with the individual patient. The doctor must see her primary role as one of safe-guarding the interests of the individual patient; anything less than this threatens both the quality and the ethical basis of health care provision.

The central problem with promoting the interests of the individual patient is that this has implications for the welfare of other patients. If an individual consumes large amounts of medical resources this could be said to be a form of indirect harm to the wider community. It is a well-accepted principle, in law at least, that individual freedom of action can be restricted on the grounds that it harms others (see Feinberg,1973). Hence, by promoting the interests of one individual, others may suffer. Clearly, there needs to be some balance struck between ensuring the welfare of the wider community of patients on the one hand and the welfare of particular individuals on the other. Within a large health care system provision should be made for the individual to exercise as much choice as possible, recognizing that this choice might have to be constrained by available resources and the needs of others.

In conclusion, when treatment decisions are being made for a particular patient the use of EBM must not eradicate an individual's clinical judgement. This is not so much a criticism of EBM rather a reminder of the role that EBM should play in medical decision making and the limitations of such a role in actual clinical encounters.

CONCLUSION

It could be argued that EBM is particularly hard to implement in general practice due to the difficulty in establishing precise diagnoses and the greater awareness of the social context of the patient. When employing EBM doctors have to begin by formulating a clinical question – a working diagnosis. In general practice this is often the hardest part of the consultation. For example, a patient presents with back pain, he has an office job and complains that sitting for a long time makes the pain worse and wants the doctor to give him a week off work. In the course of the consultation the patient mentions he is unhappy at work and that he often feels tired. The challenge here is to ascertain what the clinical question is. Is the patient depressed? Is he simply unhappy at work? Does he have something mechanically wrong with his back? In this situation, while EBM may be useful at a later stage, once the problem has been identified, initially it has little to contribute. However, these are problems that affect all areas of medicine and there are no insurmountable reasons why EBM is any less useful in general practice than hospital medicine. As long as the contribution EBM can make to clinical decision making is realistically considered, by an awareness of the uncertainty that pervades medical practice, EBM can be an invaluable tool for clinicians. As an editorial in the *BMJ* (Smith, 1997) noted, 'the information that is drowning us is biased. Whatever technique we use to try and reach the answers from the information – no matter whether it is a systematic review or grabbing the closest paper in the library – we cannot avoid that bias.' EBM simply provides the information that is brought to bear on the decision – it is not the decision itself. This should be borne in mind, lest the evaluative elements of decision making are obscured.

NOTES

1 There has been an editorial and a letter on EBM in the *Journal of Medical Ethics*, see Hope (1995) and Hughes (1996) and some articles in medical journals (Kerridge, Lowe and Henry, 1998). Naylor (1995 and 1997) has indicated some weaknesses of the approach.
2 Outcomes research is a research methodology designed to evaluate 'what works' or more technically what can be determined to be effective treatments. This is done by collecting statistical analyses of outcome data drawn from very large databases such as hospital records (or in the US insurance company records). See Gifford (1996) for an evaluation of the outcome movement and the implications for clinical judgement.
3 See also Sackett *et al.* (1991).
4 See MacNaughton (1995) for an account of the importance of anecdotes in medical practice.
5 Naylor (1995) criticizes this approach, arguing that at a fundamental level EBM is still based on opinion. Panellists who decide which research projects should be reported in journals may be 'pooling ignorance as much as distilling wisdom'.
6 For an illustration of this point, see Brazier (1992: 88).

REFERENCES

Brazier, M. (1992) *Medicine, Patients and the Law*, Harmondsworth: Penguin.

Chalmers, I. and Altman, D. (eds) (1995) *Systematic Reviews*, London, BMJ Publishing Group.

Cooper, A. B., Doig, G. S. and Sibbald, W. J. (1996) 'Pulmonary artery catheters in the critically ill: an overview of using the methodology of EBM', *Critical Care Clinician*, 12 (4): 777–94.

Davidoff, F., Case, K. and Fried, P. (1995a) 'Evidence-based medicine: why all the fuss?', *Annals of Internal Medicine*, 122(9): 727.

Davidoff, F., Haynes, B., Sackett, D. and Smith, R. (1995b) 'Evidence based medicine', *British Medical Journal*, 310: 1085.

Eysenck, H. J. (1995) 'Problems with meta-analysis', in Chalmers and Altman (eds) *Systematic Reviews*, London: BMJ Publishing Group.

Feinberg, J. (1973) *Social Philosophy*, Englewood Cliffs, NJ: Prentice-Hall.

Gifford, F. (1996) 'Outcomes research and practice guidelines', *The Hastings Center Report', March–April*: 38–44.

Grahame-Smith, D. (1995) 'Evidence based medicine: Socratic dissent', *British Medical Journal*, 310: 126–7.

Greenberg, H. M. (1994) 'Three threats to the capacity for excellence in medicine', *Annals of the New York Academy of Sciences*, 729: 8–18.

Greenhalgh, T. (1997) 'Papers that summarize other papers (systematic reviews and meta-analyses)', *British Medical Journal*, 315: 672–5.

Hope, T. (1995) 'Evidence based medicine and ethics', *Journal of Medical Ethics*, 21: 259–60.

Hopkins, A. and Solomon, J. K. (1996) 'Can contacts drive clinical care?', *British Medical Journal*, 313: 477–8.
Hughes, J. C. (1996) Letter, *Journal of Medical Ethics*, 1: 55–6.
James, B. (1993) 'Implementing practice guidelines through clinical quality improvement', *Hospital Management Review*, 3: 7.
Kerridge, I., Lowe, M. and Henry, D. (1998) 'Ethics and evidence based medicine', *British Medical Journal*, 316: 1151–3.
Kitchiner, D. and Bundred, P. (1996) 'Integrated care pathways', *Archives in Disease in Childhood*, 75: 166–8.
MacNaughton, J. (1995) 'Anecdotes and empiricism', *British Journal of General Practice*, November: 571–2.
Mulrow, C. D. (1995) 'Rational for systematic reviews', in I. Chalmers and D. Altman (eds) *Systematic Reviews*, London: BMJ Publishing Group.
Naylor, C. D. (1995) 'Grey zones of clinical practice: some limits to evidence-based medicine', *The Lancet* 345: 840–2.
Naylor, C. D. (1997) 'Meta-analysis and the meta-epidemiology of clinical research', *British Medical Journal*, 315: 617–19.
NHS Executive (1996) *Promoting Clinical Effectiveness: A Framework for action in and through the NHS*, Leeds: Department of Health.
Oxman, A. D. (1995) 'Checklist for review articles', in I. Chalmers and D. Altman (eds) *Systematic Reviews*, London: BMJ Publishing Group.
Papineau, D. (1996) *The Philosophy of Science*, Oxford: Oxford Univeristy Press.
Petitti, D. (1994) *Meta-Analysis, Decision Analysis and Cost Effectiveness: Methods for Quantitative Synthesis in Medicine*, Oxford: Oxford University Press.
Rosenberg, W. and Donald, A. (1995) 'Evidence based medicine: an approach to clinical problem solving', *British Medical Journal*, 310: 1122–6.
Sackett, D., Haynes, B., Guyatt, G. and Tugwell, P. (1991) *Clinical Epidemiology: A Basic Science for Clinical Medicine*, Boston: Little, Brown.
Segar, G. (1996) quoted in J. Tingle, 'Clinical guidelines: risk management and legal issues', *British Journal of Nursing*, 5(5).
Smith, R. (1997) 'Editor's choice', *British Medical Journal*, 315.
Suppes, P. (1979) 'The logic of clinical judgment: Bayesian and other approaches', in H. T. Engelhardt, S. F. Spicker and B. Towers (eds) *Clinical Judgment: A Critical Appraisal*, Holland: D. Reidel.
Tanenbaum, S. (1995) 'What physicians know', *The New England Journal of Medicine*, 21 October: 1268–70.
Tingle, J. (1996) 'Clinical guidelines: risk management and legal issues', *British Journal of Nursing*, 5(5): 266–7.
Tingle, J. (1997) 'Evidence based nursing and the law', *British Journal of Nursing*, 6(11): 639–41.
'Users' guide to the medical literature' (1993) *Journal of the American Medical Association*, 271.
'Users' guide to the medical literature' (1994) *Journal of the American Medical Association*, 270.

Chapter 3

Ethico-legal dilemmas within general practice

Moral indeterminacy and abstract morality

Len Doyal

It is not easy being a general practitioner in today's NHS. This is evidenced by the fact that it is becoming difficult to recruit GPs in some areas, that there are high rates of stress, divorce, alcoholism and psychiatric illness among GPs and that general practice is often accorded a relatively low status within the medical profession (McKevitt *et al.*, 1996; Caplan, 1994: 1261–3; Sutherland and Cooper, 1992: 1545–8). Contributing to these problems is the fact that GPs often face particularly demanding ethico-legal dilemmas arising from the special characteristics of the job itself. These problems concern four factors characteristic of much general practice. First, GPs have long-term relationships with patients unlike most clinicians who work in acute care. Second, GPs treat families whose members sometimes have conflicting interests and demands. Third, GPs have much less opportunity for the collaborative discussion and debate which is essential for rational decision making about ethical and legal dilemmas in medicine. And, finally, GPs often face unrealistic moral demands as regards their role as primary health carers.

In this chapter I will outline what will be deemed the 'standard' view of medical ethics and analyse why it is primarily associated with acute care in hospital. Each of the preceding characteristics of general practice will be articulated and shown to highlight the oversimplicity of the standard view. I will conclude by suggesting that the standard view may distract attention from the socio-economic circumstances of patients in ways which can make it inconsistent with the very moral goals it advocates.

RESPECT FOR AUTONOMY AS A DUTY OF CARE: THE STANDARD VIEW

Throughout the array of regulatory and advisory material published to educate doctors about their moral and legal duties of care to patients, three principles loom large. They are usually presented as setting the moral boundaries of good professional practice. Doctors should protect life and health and respect autonomy to a professional standard and they should do both in ways which are fair and just. Texts will vary as to specific definitions of these duties, but all three are usually referred to (General Medical Council 1995a and b; BMA, 1993) This chapter will concentrate on the first two.

There are few surprises about the duty to protect life and health: patients should benefit rather than be harmed from treatments duly administered. Of course, there will sometimes be the risk of harm if benefit is to be achieved. At the very least, patients must communicate private and potentially embarrassing matters about themselves and agree to be touched in ways otherwise confined only to intimate relationships. At most, patients may dramatically suffer or even die. Hence the importance of the second principle. Respect for the autonomy of competent patients ensures that they will have the final say over whether or not to accept proposed and potentially hazardous treatments. It also ensures that patients will control who has access to information which they have communicated in the process.

The principle that the autonomy of individuals should be respected is of particular importance for the present discussion. The possession of autonomy entails the ability to make choices about the future on the basis of setting goals and formulating beliefs about how to achieve them. Both the law and the medical profession accept that adult patients who have this ability also have the right to agree to what medical treatment is administered to them and for what purpose (Beauchamp and Childress, 1994: 120–88). This means that doctors (and others) have a duty to act in ways entailed by respect for this right – irrespective of their own goals, beliefs or desires. For this reason, the duty to respect autonomy can be said to trump the duty to protect life and health. If an autonomous, competent patient decides that they do not wish for their life and health to be protected, then legally and morally, there is nothing that their doctor (or, say, their relatives) can or should do to force them (Kennedy and Grubb, 1994: 334–42).

Thus the right of patients to have their autonomy respected within the clinical relationship reduces to two subsidiary rights: to consent to treatment and to confidentiality. The duty of clinicians to obtain informed consent before they proceed can only be acceptably executed if three conditions hold (Kennedy, 1992: 44–71). First, patients must be provided with accurate information about their condition, proposed treatments and risks. How much information must be disclosed for consent to be legally valid is a complex issue, and it will not be considered here (Mason *et al.*, 1994: 237–47). Second, patients must be competent to consent. Legally, this entails that they can understand, remember, reason about and believe relevant clinical information about themselves (*Re C*, 1993: 77–83). And third, patients must not be coerced into making decisions to have treatment which they would otherwise reject. Their choices must be identifiable with them and no one else (*Re T*, 1992: 46–68).

The duty to protect the confidentiality of patients is a clear extension of the more general duty to respect their autonomy. Generally, privacy is of the utmost importance for individuals (Doyal, 1997a: 1–21). It is a precondition for the intimacy associated with primary relationships which themselves are morally defined by trust – the belief by all parties that what is deemed private by any of them will not be made public. Successful clinical relationships are possible only if patients are willing to communicate intimate details of their symptoms and other personal information. This is unlikely to happen if they believe that others might be given access to such information without their consent. Professionally, any unjustified breach of confidence can incur the most serious censure. Practically, the duty to respect confidentiality is focused on obtaining the patient's consent for disclosures to any third party not directly involved with their clinical care (see Chapter 4).

The right to confidentiality is, however, more morally and legally qualified than the right to consent to treatment (McHale, 1994). There are a number of circumstances where doctors are professionally and/or legally obligated to disclose information to others, irrespective of the wishes of patients (Kennedy and Grubb, 1994: 644–71). These pertain to situations where respect for confidentiality might pose potential harm to others. For example, doctors must make such disclosures if patients have been in an automobile accident and the police request information about them. Doctors also have the discretion to make disclosures if they believe that the actions of patients may lead to the serious harm of specific individuals of whom the clinician has knowledge.

There are a number of moral justifications which are usually given for placing so much professional and legal emphasis on respect for autonomy within medicine. The least convincing are utilitarian ones which justify such respect by reference to the greater individual or aggregate happiness to which it will lead. The problem with this argument is that it can also be used to defend not respecting the autonomy of patients. After all, obtaining proper informed consent can also be distressing in relation to the communication of information about prognosis and risks (Doyal, 1997b: 1107–11). Further, not informing significant other carers about the clinical problems of some patients may lead to them being denied care and concern which they would otherwise receive.

A better moral justification for the importance of respect for autonomy is that it is this attribute which gives humans their particular moral status. Animals cannot plan and choose in the same way so that respect for human dignity and for autonomy become inseparable. Equally, to the degree that we would wish for our own autonomy to be respected in clinical circumstances – and the evidence is that most people do – then it is irrational not to uphold the principle of such respect, even if in certain circumstances unhappiness might result. We can never know for sure when illness may befall us. Without support for the equal right of everyone to exercise as much control over their medical destiny as is practically possible, we cannot ensure such control will not be taken from us. If the right to respect for autonomy is taken seriously, the fact that this may sometimes create distress will cut little moral ice.

Thus, according to the standard view, the moral and legal principles governing respect for autonomy in clinical medicine are clear and there is widespread agreement that they can be philosophically defended (Gillon, 1985: 111–25). This being said, it is also recognized that far from solving all ethico-legal dilemmas within medicine, the enunciation and acceptance of these principles itself poses problems when they are applied to cases where their correct interpretation is not obvious. Unfortunately (or fortunately for medical ethicists) there can also be circumstances in which there is considerable disagreement about what good clinical practice entails in practice.

For example, as regards informed consent, clinicians often disagree about the amount of information about prognosis and risk to which patients are morally and legally entitled (Letters, *BMJ*, 1997: 1477–83; 247–54). They can also disagree about the circumstances in which the likelihood of harm warrants a breach of confidentiality – for example, when known actual or potential criminal activity which could harm others should be reported to a third party whatever the views of the patient involved (McHale, 1994: 71–99). No appeal to the duty of care can solve the problem of who is right in such circumstances since it is the interpretation of the principle of respect for autonomy which itself poses the problem.

For this reason, the standard view of medical ethics recognizes that good clinical practice also requires procedural principles for the resolution of conflict about such interpretations. Debate is inevitable in the face of moral indeterminacy concerning autonomy and will often require compromise. If decisions are to be as rational as possible under the circumstances, health care teams need to conduct debate in accordance with specific procedures designed to optimize collective reason (Doyal and Gough, 1991: 116–26). Such teams should ensure, for example, that arbitrary vested interests are not allowed to determine which interpretation will be put into practice. Of equal importance will be provision for adequate representation of expertise relevant to the best available solution to the problem at hand. If those who have something positive to contribute to debate are disenfranchised then decision making will be sub-optimal.

INFORMED CONSENT IN GENERAL PRACTICE: THE MORAL COMPLEXITY OF RESPECT FOR CRITICAL AUTONOMY

The degree to which the standard view of medical ethics is linked to the practice of acute medicine within the hospital sector should be clear. Here, the pretence is that patients are either competent to give adequate consent to treatment on the basis of relevant information or they are not. Patients either are autonomous or they are not. If they are, respect for their autonomy within hospital usually occurs in what might be called a 'slice of time' – the time it takes to attempt to communicate information about proposed treatments and for patients to provide or refuse consent. Unless they have manifest psychiatric symptoms of incompetence, the presumption will be that such patients are capable of providing autonomous consent. Respect for their autonomy means that their decision will be accepted by their hospital clinician – even if it conflicts with what is perceived to be in their best clinical interests. On the standard view of what such respect should entail, rejection of such decisions or attempts to coerce patients into agreement are regarded as the unacceptable face of clinical paternalism.

If we begin with informed consent, however, a distance quickly becomes apparent between good general practice and the standard view of respect for autonomy. Unlike hospital doctors working in the acute sector, moral life is more difficult for general practitioners. Most patients who are asked to give explicit consent to treatment in hospital are strangers to the doctors who obtain it. Good GPs, however, know their patients well – their intellectual and emotional strengths, weaknesses and personal awareness of both. They are given an entry into the private lives of their patients over long periods of time which creates a special moral relationship with them (Heath, 1995: 23–46). They may not be their patients' friends but the moral texture – the trust, intimacy and sustained character – of the relationship is analogous to that of friendship. Therefore, the patterns of diagnosis and treatment typical of good general practice are far removed from the slices of time and anonymity often associated with formally obtaining consent for treatment in a hospital environment.

As regards respect for autonomy, the crucial moral difference between hospital doctors and GPs is best illustrated not by the right to agree to treatment but by the right to refuse it. Thus when doctors in hospital respect the right of patients to refuse treatment and to damage or even kill themselves in the process, they do so in the secure knowledge that they will probably never see them or their relatives again. GPs have no such luxury. Their patients who are uncooperative – either as regards treatment or prevention – continue to present themselves and their problems for further review (Christie and Hoffmaster, 1986: 146–60). And they do so against the background of the emotional bonds generated between themselves, their families and their GPs over long periods. Therefore, within general practice the potential conflict between the duty to protect life and health and to respect autonomy can repeatedly come home with a vengeance rarely experienced in sustained ways in the acute hospital sector. This highlights the moral over-simplicity of the way these duties are often talked about (Doyal, 1987: 1579–82).

As an illustration, let us take an example of an uncooperative patient – say, 33-year-old Mrs Jones – who is a single parent to two young children and who works as a secretary. She has asthma but continues to smoke. Imagine the following clinical encounter: the patient complains about her increasingly frequent attacks and her difficulty in controlling them with her current medication. The GP asks whether or not she is continuing to smoke and she confirms this – although 'she has dramatically cut down' – despite the attempts which he has already made to help her understand why tobacco poses such a danger for someone with her condition. What should a good GP do in this situation?

If we return to the standard model of respect for autonomy, the answer is clear. The patient has made her choice – to refuse to heed his clinical advice. He should respect it and the autonomy which informed it. It is, after all, her body and her right to do with it as she sees fit. Or is it? Does she have no obligation toward her future self – the person she will become when the damaging results of her smoking perhaps become irreversible? What about her responsibilities toward her children, for whom the GP is also clinically responsible? Even if we leave the dangers of passive smoking out of the equation, her children are dependent on her and in this respect alone they will be negatively affected by the continuation of smoking related illness. The same questions pose themselves, of course, as regards a wide range of uncooperative and self-damaging behaviour by patients with other chronic conditions – not to mention even more common examples of non-cooperation concerning drugs, diet and exercise (Stockwell and Schulz, 1992: 8283–95; McGavock *et al.*, 1996).

Many GPs do not acknowledge the professional appropriateness of automatically accepting such an ostensible manifestation of autonomy as Mrs Jones' choice to reject the advice offered. They recognize – at least intuitively – that autonomy is more complicated than the standard model suggests (Toon, 1987: 502–4). We have seen that the criteria for judging levels of autonomy for providing informed consent are minimal to say the least and linked more to the provision of acute hospital rather than primary care. They are designed to detect those who are incapable of making an informed decision about an immediate therapeutic intervention, not those who in fact are making competent decisions about lifestyle or other aspects of long-term medical care – albeit decisions which are not in their own best interests or those who rely upon them.

To the degree that the practice of obtaining consent only conforms to such minimal standards, then it is clear that the autonomy of the patients concerned may be low. Then agreement to treatment or to follow other clinical advice may not be really informed at all. To pretend otherwise – to regard autonomy as a thing which patients either fully possess or do not with respect to the task of consenting to treatment – is to do them and their clinicians a disservice (Doyal, 1990: 1–16).

A better approach is to regard autonomy as a variable rather than a thing or a fixed set of attributes. The value of the variable will then be dependent on the values of three subsidiary variables: understanding, emotional confidence and social opportunity. Patients cannot give reasonable levels of agreement to treatment unless they properly understand related information (including correctly being able to answer questions about it if asked), are confident enough to act on whatever choice they then make and are helped to avoid social constraints in their lives which lead to poor levels of understanding and confidence (Doyal and Gough, 1991: 59–75 and 180–90).

To pretend that consent which accepts low values of these variables can reasonably be called 'informed' is no more than a medico-legal artefact designed to enable clinicians to do little more than identify a choice with an individual patient (Faden and Beauchamp, 1986: 298–336). In the hospital setting of acute care, this does not necessarily present as a moral problem because patients either agree to treatment, whatever the degree of offered information, or they refuse and this is accepted with little further exploration.

This is why GPs who have forged long-term clinical relationships with their patients may quite legitimately not respect their autonomy in the minimal sense which has been outlined. GPs may rightly question clinical decisions by patients which they believe not to be in their best interests. A minimally autonomous choice is not one which is necessarily educated or confident. Therefore, GPs do a disservice to patients whose educational, emotional and social weaknesses are well known to them if they automatically accept their self-damaging decisions. Rather, they should do their best to help patients to enhance the levels of autonomy which inform their choices about health care and lifestyle, wherever this is practically possible. When this becomes the moral goal of respecting the autonomy of patients then the acceptance of any minimally competent choice no longer counts as a morally acceptable version of such respect. What is acceptable is trying to help patients to understand why what they want is not necessarily what they need, including providing access to counselling about how to develop the confidence and motivation to act on such understanding (Toon, 1994: 31–6).

GPs may employ a host of stratagems to provide such help. Thus Mrs Jones' GP may in a range of ways – including perhaps a certain amount of coercion – encourage her to understand the damage that she is doing to her health and the present and future well being of her children. The GP's long-term care for her may reinforce his or her concern and fire his or her motivation to help her to help herself. This may involve the provision of further information about the dangers which tobacco particularly poses for her and persistent emotional pressure on her to try to understand it and to consider appropriate counselling.

Similar considerations apply to non-cooperative behaviour as regards other chronic illnesses – the same caring struggle to help patients to optimize what has been called their 'critical autonomy': their potential to move beyond their first order preferences to more educated and confident second order preferences. We would and should think morally less of GPs who did otherwise (Doyal and Gough, 1991: 59–69, 187–90; Dworkin, 1988: 20).

Yet deciding when it is appropriate not to respect first order unreflective choice and to insist on more informed and reflective second order choice is not easy for GPs. On the one hand, they may appreciate the degree to which they may be wrong about the level of deliberation which has informed the choices of patients (Wright, 1993: 909–10). For example, Mrs Jones may be well aware of the dangers which smoking poses to her and her children. She may also understand the degree to which her habit is reinforced by the stresses associated with her personal and professional life and have calculated that her access to tobacco is for the moment more important for her successful negotiation of both spheres. In this context, she may correctly understand that at present it may be in her own and others' best interests for her to smoke. If her GP goes too far in his attempts to dissuade her – given that her decision is an optimally informed one – then he may irreparably harm the very clinical relationship which in the longer term may still help her to give up tobacco.

On the other hand – and with the preceding dilemma in mind – the moral and medico-legal fact remains that provided patients are competent, even their first order autonomous choices trump those of their GPs. For the reasons which have been given, paternalism can be justified in the face of self-damaging decisions by patients with low levels of autonomy. However, the acceptable boundaries of paternalism remain with the strict duty to acknowledge that, at any point in time, patients have the right to reject clinical advice. Once it is clear that this really is what they are doing 'it matters not whether the reasons for the refusal were rational or irrational, unknown or even non-existent' (Re *T*, 1992: 62).

Yet GPs have to judge the point of refusal at which further debate *is* both pointless and morally irresponsible. It is not easy. Therefore, the implications of the standard view of medical ethics as regards respect for individual autonomy are often unclear within general practice and this creates dilemmas not so often faced by hospital doctors.

CONFIDENTIALITY AND GENERAL PRACTICE: THE MORAL BOUNDARIES OF ACCEPTABLE DISCLOSURE OF INFORMATION TO OTHERS

Things become no better for GPs when we turn to their duty to respect the right of patients to control access to private information communicated within the confines of the clinical relationship. We have seen the degree to which the standard view of medical ethics places great stress on the moral importance of respect for the right to confidentiality, emphasizing its link to the relationship of trust so crucial for successful clinical relationships. It has also been indicated that the right of patients to confidentiality is much more qualified than that to consent to treatment – there is more scope for breaching it within morally and legally acceptable boundaries.

The primary reason for such qualification concerns the nature of human rights themselves. Among other things, rights can be regarded as claims on others who accept the duty to honour the claim (Steiner, 1994: 59–73). Such claims will hardly be regarded by others as reasonable if they know that they might seriously harm themselves through respecting them. In other words, our rights stop at the point at which they threaten serious harm to others. It is this moral belief which is behind many of the breaches of confidence which are deemed acceptable within the practice of good medicine (Doyal, 1997a). Thus, in a variety of circumstances, the interests of the public are seen as trumping the right of the patient to confidentiality – sometimes so much as to compel the clinician to breach it (e.g. the prevention of terrorism) and sometimes to enable such a breach provided that the clinician deems it warranted (e.g. disclosure of information to the police about a suspected murderer) (Kennedy and Grubb, 1994: 644–71).

Yet despite the potentially qualified character of the right to confidentiality, in most clinical practice the duty to respect it remains of great importance and is stressed by the regulatory institutions of medicine (General Medical Council, 1995b). Within the practice of acute hospital care, the implementation of respect for such rights is again relatively straightforward. As with informed consent, professional duties towards patients are discharged in a slice of time where the patient per se remains the focus of moral responsibility.

According to the standard view, good practice entails the communication of information about competent patients to others only with their explicit or implied consent. In the case of incompetent patients, information should only be communicated to those who are not involved in the patients' care – such as relatives – in two circumstances. On the one hand, it might be necessary in the best interests of patients to acquire information about them through discussions with others about their condition and proposed treatment. On the other hand, preparations for care at home or elsewhere may need to be made when patients leave hospital. This too may necessitate some disclosure of information in their best interests, again, on a 'need to know basis' (Montgomery, 1997: 255–6).

If relatives or friends are unhappy about the levels of disclosure deemed appropriate in hospital, they may complain. However, there is little else they can do. Clinicians know that it is highly likely that they will have no further contact after patients have been discharged. Indeed, even in those rare circumstances where clinicians must or may breach confidentiality, this lack of further contact will make any disclosure relatively painless. Patients who enter hospital as strangers will often be discharged with little detailed and intimate knowledge gained about their personal lives.

Things are not so straightforward for GPs. They are clinically responsible not just for individuals but for individuals in families. Family members may have the interests of each other at heart or may be in conflict with each other. In most circumstances, it is reasonable to assume that relatives emotionally and materially care for each other and primarily wish for benefit to result from clinical care (Nelson and Nelson, 1995: 55–118). However, it would be dangerous to assume that this is always so (Brazier, 1992: 448). In either case, through their desire to support or to harm, relatives can place enormous pressure on GPs to reveal information about the diagnosis and treatment of individual family members – pressure which can sometimes be difficult to resist (Lako and Lindenthal, 1990: 167–70).

The primary reason for this difficulty returns us to the other key difference between general practitioners and many hospital doctors. Not only are GPs responsible for treating members of the same families, they have long-term relationships with them all. In practice this means that each family member will know that the GP has information about other family members that they may wish to know for morally acceptable or unacceptable reasons. In attempting to discover such information, they can arrange to see their GP for a host of other reasons and the GP knows that they can do so – time and time again. As a family member, they can even request confidential information directly, playing on the generally held belief that family members want to help and not harm each other.

The pressure to breach confidentiality can be even greater when GPs know for sure that through maintaining it they may well harm the very patient whom they have a duty of care to protect. Often it genuinely is the case that relatives need information about the clinical condition of patients in order to provide them with appropriate emotional and material support. Their requests for information can be what GPs know are genuine expressions of concern and care. When this is combined with lack of certainty for whatever reason about what patients want their relatives to know, it is hardly surprising that sometimes GPs do collude with relatives in ways which constitute a technical breach of confidentiality (Lako and Lindenthal, 1991: 153–7).

Equally, we have seen that circumstances exist where disclosure of clinical information can be justified to avoid harm to others. This is usually when the risk of such harm is serious – death or permanent and irreversible injury, for example (Montgomery, 1997: 557–61). Yet how serious is serious? Because they are family doctors, GPs will often know of the harm that one member is inflicting on another, without the latter necessarily understanding the extent of this. As a result, family members may be unable to take appropriate steps to protect themselves or other family members. It is now commonplace that if the potential threat is serious and physical then GPs do have the discretion to disclose – having indicated to the patient that this is their intention. But what if the threat is still serious but emotional – caused, for example, by a patient refusing to reveal clinical information about themselves which other members of the family need in order to plan their future or possibly to protect themselves? If my right to confidentiality stops at the point at which respect for it harms members of my family, in what physical and emotional circumstances should GPs recognize this fact and disclose accordingly?

There are no easy answers to these questions. What is important is the recognition that they constitute an ethical dilemma facing GPs more often than hospital doctors and that this derives from their unique and long-term relationships with their patients – both as individuals and as members of families. Against the background of the recognized scope for discretion in breaching confidentiality in some circumstances and of the legitimate interests of many families in erstwhile confidential information about individual members, GPs should clarify and make public their policies of disclosure of such information. Then families can understand the range of questions which cannot be answered without the consent of the patients concerned. Such statements should also make clear to patients the stress that can be caused by concerned relatives who inquire about clinical circumstances of other family members. Competent patients should always be asked their views about who they wish to be given information about what and these views should be included in their clinical record.

In many situations, patients may well be happy for relatives to be given private information and, if invited, explicitly consent to it (Benson and Britten, 1996: 729–31). However, if they opt for confidentiality then – subject to the accepted qualifications for mandatory or discretionary disclosure – this must be respected, despite the sustained pressures from other family members which this may impose on the doctor. It is the character of this pressure – combined with the detailed knowledge of, and long-term relationship with, such family members – that makes respect for confidentiality so difficult for many GPs. When competent patients are not given the opportunity to decide who in their family should have access to information about them which would otherwise be confidential, it should always be assumed that their privacy should be respected. In a recent interesting study, this is precisely what patients themselves indicated that they wished (Benson and Britten, 1996)

MORAL INDETERMINACY, COLLECTIVE DECISION MAKING AND THE ABSURDITIES OF ABSTRACT MORALITY

The final reason why GPs can face more moral pressure than many hospital doctors, especially in the acute sector, relates to their need to interpret substantive moral principles in relation to individual cases. We have seen that the acceptance of orthodox formulations of the duties of care will not necessarily resolve clinical or moral dilemmas. In hard cases where the correct resolution is unclear, collective decision making can be important in achieving a resolution. If the solution to the problem is unclear and compromise probable, it is best to have as many voices as possible to contribute to the solution and share responsibility for it. To do otherwise is to rely on the potential arbitrariness of only one opinion.

Hospital doctors are much better placed to implement such collective decision making than GPs. The social and professional organization of hospital medicine incorporates the importance of group discussion and regular review of clinical and moral decisions. Often, GPs do not have similar opportunities for such collective deliberation. They and they alone must make judgements about which they may not be completely confident – and they may be mistaken (Newman, 1996: 71–5). Single practitioners obviously lack such opportunities. In many group practices, partners do not meet regularly for collective debate and discussion about clinical and ethical matters and practice meetings can too often be focused only on business or management issues.

The stressfulness of clinical isolation can be attenuated by the opportunity for referral. Where GPs are genuinely unsure or where the condition of the patient is too acute to risk error, there is the option of either seeking a specialized opinion or even placing the patient in hospital. The same cannot be said, however, for the difficult and often indeterminate ethical dilemmas faced by GPs. Here, there is no one to whom the patient can be referred and, often, no one with the relevant training and experience to debate the pros and cons of related moral and legal arguments. This is especially serious given the degree and complexity of some of the dilemmas described above.

The situation facing GPs working in deprived areas can be even worse. We have established that it is the duty of the good GP to try to enhance the autonomy of patients – particularly those who are clinically uncooperative in ways which potentially harm themselves or other members of their families. The related ethico-legal problems which have been outlined are difficult enough with patients who are highly educated, emotionally secure and surrounded by a range of social opportunities which enhance their autonomy. The difficulties increase for GPs with patients from deprived socio-economic backgrounds, who are poorly educated and may be emotionally brutalized by their circumstances. Here the danger is of allowing talk of the GP's duty of care to respect autonomy to be reduced to a moral abstraction which sounds good in principle but is impossible to deliver. For what does it mean to argue that, in such circumstances, GPs have a moral duty to help their patients to optimize their autonomy against the background of their environmental deficits – at least as regards the clinical encounter itself (Doyal, 1995: 55–62)?

Some reasonable demarcation of professional responsibility is necessary, along with a realistic appraisal of what is and is not achievable with patients as regards education and counselling. However, there are few opportunities to discuss such matters with colleagues and little constructive advice is forthcoming either from within the medical profession or from moral commentators on it. It can be extremely frustrating for GPs to be in a situation where they are expected to do their best to respect and nourish the critical autonomy of patients during their consultations while knowing that they will return to the very environment which helped to minimize their autonomy in the first place.

So what should be done to improve matters? GPs should have regular fora where such problems can be discussed and where responsibility for strategies for their optimal resolution can be shared. Yet the importance of collective reason should not be overestimated. Many of the moral indeterminacies which have been described will never receive any adequate resolution at the level of general practice because their origins extend far beyond it – especially those relating to the socio-economic and cultural background of patients.

What will not help in dealing with the moral dilemmas posed is more abstract moralizing. The danger is that the standard model of medical ethics – an ethics which we have seen is often divorced from the everyday realities of general practice – can undermine the feeling of worth and moral integrity of GPs. If the advocacy of moral and professional virtue in general practice leads to this result then its price will be too high (Toon, forthcoming). We must temper our moral ideals to the social and professional realities within which we expect GPs to serve others and to survive themselves.

CONCLUSION

This chapter has argued that GPs often have to face tougher ethico-legal decisions than their hospital counterparts, especially in the acute sector. Within hospital medicine, respect for the principle of autonomy – of informed consent and of confidentiality – can be relatively straightforward. Such respect occurs in a slice of time, divorced from the ongoing narrative of the lives of both patients and clinicians. This means that hospital doctors can often escape with applying low educational standards to consent for and refusal of treatment. Also, they can usually implement the principle of confidentiality without having to confront the pressures which professional relationships with other family members can pose.

We have seen that GPs are not so fortunate. The long-term relationships which they have with their patients – as individuals and family members – demand the goal of engendering critical autonomy, at times at the expense of respect for minimal autonomy. These relationships also entail living with the moral tensions within families and coping with the pressures which families can place on them to breach confidentiality. Hospital doctors do sometimes face similar issues but not nearly so regularly or systematically.

It has been argued that one important way of dealing with the moral indeterminacies encountered within general practice is for GPs to try to create more opportunity for collective discussion and debate about such matters. If, in the face of such indeterminacy, moral compromise is inevitable, it is crucial for it to be reached as the result of optimally rational decision making. Finally, to divorce medical ethics and moral character from attempts to get improvements in the living and working conditions of patients will undermine the goals of good general practice and the moral principles which inform it.

ACKNOWLEDGEMENT

Many thanks to Lesley Doyal, Peter Toon, Iona Heath, Brian Hurwitz and, especially, Richard Mitchell.

REFERENCES

Beauchamp, T. and Childress, J. (1994) *Principles of Biomedical Ethics*, New York: Oxford University Press.

Benson, J. and Britten, N. (1996) 'Respecting the autonomy of cancer patients when talking with their relatives: qualitative analysis of semistructured interviews with patients', *British Medical Journal*, 313: 729–31.

Brazier, M. (1992) *Medicine, Patients and the Law*, Harmondsworth: Penguin.

British Medical Association, Ethics, Science and Information Division (1993) *Medical Ethics Today: Its Practice and Philosophy*, London: BMA.

British Medical Journal (1997) Letters on informed consent, 314: 1477–83 and 315: 247–54.

Caplan, R.P. (1994) 'Stress, anxiety and depression in hospital consultants, general practitioners, and senior health service managers', *British Medical Journal*, 309: 1261–3.

Christie, R.J. and Hoffmaster, C.B. (1986) *Ethical Issues in Family Medicine*, New York, Oxford University Press.

Davis, H. and Fallowfield, L. (1991) *Counselling and Communication in Health Care*, Chichester: Wiley.

Doyal, L. (1987) 'General practice, chronic care and the treatment of difficult patients', *The Practitioner*, November: 1579–82.

Doyal, L. (1990) 'Medical ethics and moral indeterminacy', *Journal of Law and Society*, 17(1): 1–16.

Doyal, L. (1995) 'Medical ethics and good health care: the ideology of individualism', in F. Mercado, L. Martinez and L. Silva (eds) *La Medicina al Final del Milenio*, Guadalajara: University of Guadalajara Press.

Doyal, L. (1997a) 'Human need and the right of patients to privacy', *Journal of Contemporary Health Law and Policy*, 14: 1–21.

Doyal, L. (1997b) 'Journals should not publish research to which patients have not given fully informed consent – with three exceptions', *British Medical Journal*, 314: 1107–11.

Doyal, L. and Gough, I. (1991) *A Theory of Human Need*, London: Macmillan.

Dworkin, G. (1988) *The Theory and Practice of Autonomy*, Cambridge: Cambridge University Press.

Faden, R. and Beauchamp, T. (1986) *A History and Theory of Informed Consent*, New York: Oxford University Press.

General Medical Council (1995a) *Duties of a Doctor*, London: General Medical Council.

General Medical Council (1995b) *Confidentiality*, London: General Medical Council.

Gillon, R. (1985) 'Autonomy and consent', in M. Lockwood (ed.) *Moral Dilemmas in Modern Medicine,* Oxford: Oxford University Press.

Heath, I. (1995) *The Mystery of General Practice*, London: Nuffield Provincial Hospitals Trust.

Kennedy, I. (1992) 'Consent to treatment: the capable person', in C. Dyer (ed.) *Doctors, Patients and the Law*, Oxford: Blackwell.

Kennedy, I. and Grubb, A. (1994) *Medical Law: Text with Materials*, London: Butterworths.

Lako, C.J. and Lindenthal, J.J. (1990) 'Confidentiality in medical practice', *Journal of Family Practitioners*, 31: 167–70.

Lako, C.J. and Lindenthal, J.J. (1991) 'The management of confidentiality in general medical practice: a comparative study in the USA and the Netherlands', *Social Science and Medicine*, 32: 153–7.

McGavock, H., Britten, N. and Weinman, J. (1996) *A Review of the Literature on Drug Adherence*, London: Royal Pharmacological Society of Great Britain.

McHale, J. (1994) *Medical Confidentiality and Legal Privilege*, London: Routledge.

McKevitt, C., Morgan, M., Simpson, J. and Holland, W. (1996) *Doctor's Health and Needs for Services*, London: Nuffield Provincial Hospital Trust.

Mason, J.K. and McCall Smith, R.A. (1994) *Law and Medical Ethics*: London, Butterworths.

Montgomery, J. (1997) *Health Care Law*, Oxford: Oxford University Press.

Nelson, H.L. and Nelson, J.L. (1995) *The Patient in the Family*, New York: Routledge.

Newman, M.C. (1996) 'The emotional impact of mistakes on family physicians', *Archive of Family Medicine*, 5(2): 71–5.

Re C (1993) Butterworths Medico-Legal Reports, 15: 77–83.

Re T (1992) Butterworths Medico-Legal Reports, 9: 46–68.

Steiner, H. (1994) *An Essay on Rights*, Oxford: Blackwell.

Stockwell, M.L. and Schulz, R.M. (1992) 'Patient compliance – an overview', *Journal of Clinical Pharmacology and Therapeutics*, 17: 283–95.

Sutherland, V.J. and Cooper, C.L. (1992) 'Job stress, satisfaction, and mental health among general practitioners before and after introduction of new contract', *British Medical Journal*, 304: 1545–8.

Toon, P. (1994) *What is Good General Practice*, London: Royal College of General Practitioners.

Toon, P. (forthcoming) *The virtuous practitioner.*

Toon, P.D. (1987) 'Promoting prevention and patient autonomy', *Journal of the Royal Society of Medicine*, 80(26): 502–4.

Wright, E.C. (1993) 'Non-compliance – or how many aunts has Matilda?', *Lancet*, 342: 909–10.

Chapter 4

The general practitioner and confidentiality

Jean McHale

Confidentiality has long been part of the ethical codes of the medical profession. From the days of the Hippocratic Oath to the ethical code of the General Medical Council today doctors have been exhorted to maintain the confidentiality of their patient information. There are two main reasons why it can be regarded as being of importance. The first is that it is necessary because unless it is assured then patients will not be willing to come forward for treatment. This is an argument forcibly used in the context of certain medical conditions, for example venereal disease and HIV/AIDS. In *X* v *Y* ([1988] 2 All ER 648), Rose J. stated that

> In the long run preservation of confidentiality is the only way of securing public health: otherwise doctors will be discredited as a source of education, for future patients will not come forward if doctors are going to squeal on them. Consequently confidentiality is vital to secure public as well as private health, for unless those affected come forward they cannot be counselled and self-treatment does not provide the best care: opportunistic infections such as a shortness of breath and signs of disease in the nervous system ... are better detected and responded to by observation, investigation and management in hospital (at 653).

The second argument advanced for the maintenance of confidentiality is that of privacy (McHale, 1993). In the common law jurisdictions the right to privacy have been only relatively recently recognized. In the US in a leading article in 1890 two eminent academic commentators, Warren and Brandise, spoke of the right to be left alone (Warren and Brandise, 1890). The notion of privacy encompasses protection of access to one's own personal information and one part of such control is control over personal information which individuals may regard as 'confidential'. Today privacy rights are commonly enshrined in human rights declarations such as the European Convention on Human Rights (Article 8). This principle has been affirmed in the recent European Convention on Human Rights and Biomedicine (Article 10). While the UK has been a party to the European Convention of Human Rights for many years, we have not had our own home grown Bill of Rights akin to that of the European Convention until now. The Human Rights Act 1998 will require the courts to give effect to legislation in a manner compatible with the European Convention on Human Rights and it is likely that there will be increased litigation in this area on human rights issues, such as a right to privacy in the future.

Nonetheless, privacy rights are rarely regarded in absolute terms. They are habitually qualified by other considerations, so for example, in the context of the European Convention on Human Rights, Article 8 provides that:

1 Everyone shall have a right to privacy of home, family life and correspondence.
2 There shall be no interference by a public authority with this right save such as is in accordance with the law and is necessary in a democratic society in the interests of public safety, the economic well being of the country, for the prevention of disorder or crime, for the protection of health or morals or for the protection of the rights and freedoms of others.

Confidentiality is also not regarded as absolute in its nature. The General Medical Council recognizes a series of exceptions (GMC, 1995) and English law does not regard the obligation as absolute in its nature, as we shall see below.

The importance of confidentiality is reflected both in law and in health care practice (McHale and Fox, 1997). However, the operation of the principle may frequently prove problematic. In this chapter I examine the basis on which health care information is required to be maintained as confidential, the circumstances in which it can be legitimately disclosed and some of the difficult dilemmas surrounding confidentiality which may affect the general practitioner in her practice.

CONFIDENTIALITY: A LEGAL OBLIGATION

English law requires the general practitioner to maintain the confidentiality of patient information. However, there are only very limited situations in which a doctor is required by statute to maintain patient confidentiality. One such situation is in the context of venereal disease (NHS Venereal Disease Regulations SI 1974 No. 29). Another is contained in the Human Fertilisation and Embryology Act 1990 which makes it a criminal offence for unauthorized disclosure to be made of information concerning infertility treatment protected under this legislation (section 31). (The statute contains a number of exceptions sanctioning disclosure.) It is notable that in both cases the statutory provision is safeguarding health care information which is regarded as being particularly sensitive in nature. The patient with venereal disease may feel inhibited in seeking treatment without the promise that disclosure will not be made; the couple who are infertile may want to ensure that the confidentiality of such information is maintained to prevent embarrassment and distress. But such statutory protection is limited. The general safeguards for confidential information provided in English law derive from case law developed in the courts and are contained in what is known as the equitable remedy of breach of confidence. If information is entrusted to a health care professional in a situation in which that information is the subject of an obligation of confidence expressed or implied then, if the health care professional makes an unauthorized disclosure of that information, the patient may begin legal proceedings. The usual remedy here will be an injunction to stop further disclosure of the information.

However, this legal obligation of confidence is not absolute. First, the patient may herself sanction disclosure through giving express consent to disclosure. Second, information may be disclosed in situations in which it is in the 'public interest' to do so. As was confirmed by the House of Lords in *AG* v *Guardian Newspapers* (No. 2) ([1988] 3 All ER 545), the obligation of confidentiality must be balanced against the requirement that disclosure is in the public interest. There is no one comprehensive definition of what precisely constitutes the 'public interest'. As we shall see below, in breach of confidence cases concerning health care information the courts have taken note of the statements of confidentiality and agreed exceptions recognized by the General Medical Council (e.g. *W* v *Egdell* [1990] 1 All ER 835).

DISCLOSURE WITH PATIENT CONSENT AND IN THE NEED OF PATIENT CARE

In relation to patient information protected under the equitable remedy of breach of confidence, patient consent is necessary before disclosure is made, save where disclosure is in the public interest. But the extent to which an express consent to disclosure should be given in every situation has been questioned. In their guidance paper, *The Protection and Use of Patient Information*, the Department of Health stated that:

> 2.5 It is neither practicable nor necessary to seek a patient's (or other informant's) specific consent each time information needs to be passed on for a particular purpose. The public expects the NHS, often in conjunction with other agencies, to respond effectively to its needs; it can do so only if it has the necessary information. Therefore, an essential feature of the relationship between patients and the NHS is the need for patients to be fully informed of the uses to which information about them may be put:(see section 3 and paragraph 4.4).

How far this implied consent necessarily corresponds to patient expectation may be questioned. This also makes it important that patients should be aware of the basis on which their information is liable to be disclosed. The Department of Health guidance goes on to state that,

> 3.1 All NHS bodies must have an active policy for informing patients of the kind of purposes for which information about them is collected and the categories of people or organisations to which information may need to be passed. Where other bodies are providing services for or in conjunction with the NHS, those concerned must be aware of each other's information policies.
>
> 3.2 Subject to some important common elements …, the precise arrangements for informing patients are for local decision, taking account of views expressed by community health councils, local patient groups, staff and agencies with which the NHS body is in close contact. However, those concerned, should bear in mind that:
>
> i as a general rule, patients should be told how information would be used before they are asked to provide it and must have the opportunity to discuss any aspects that are special to their treatment or circumstances;
>
> ii advice must be presented in a convenient form and be available both for general purposes and before a particular programme of care and treatment begins.

3.3 Methods of providing advice include;

- leaflets enclosed with patients' appointment letters or provided when prescriptions are dispensed;
- GP practice leaflets and/or notification on initial registration with a GP;
- routinely providing patients with necessary information as part of care planning;
- identifying someone to provide further information if patients want it.

The purposes for which information can be disclosed include management purposes and also extend to a 'need to know' basis, as stated in paragraph 2.6 of the guidance which includes NHS purposes where:

> the recipient needs the information because he or she is or may be concerned with the patient's care and treatment (or that of another patient whose health may be affected by the condition of the original patient such as a blood or organ donor).

In such a situation the recipient, e.g. doctor or nurse, would most likely be subject to a professional ethical obligation along with a stipulation to maintain confidentiality contained in the contract of employment.

The GMC, in a statement on confidentiality issued in 1995, provides that information may be disclosed in the public interest in limited situations:

> Disclosure may be necessary in the public interest where a failure to disclose information may expose the patient or others to risk of death or serious harm. In such circumstances you should disclose information promptly to an appropriate person or authority.
>
> (GMC, 1995: Clause 18)

Although disclosure may be made in the public interest, that does not equate with general availability of information. Instead it is the case that information should be disclosed to persons for whom it is in the public interest to know, rather than members of the public who find the information interesting (*Lion Laboratories* v *Evans* [1984] 2 All ER 417). Where disclosure is made this should be limited to those to whom disclosure is truly necessary. It also appears that 'public interest' here does not refer to harm to the public as a whole and may be sufficient if the harm in question relates to one specific individual (Jones, 1990).

Difficult issues remain. In determining the public interest the court has indicated that it will be prepared to take note of the guidelines issued by the General Medical Council on the subject. However, these guidelines themselves still leave much discretion in the hands of the doctor in determining whether or not to disclose. For example, while most would agree that, faced with a patient who is clearly psychopathic and who has informed the GP that he has killed in the past and intends to kill again, disclosure would be justified, disclosure in relation to other crimes actual/anticipated are less clear. An illustration of circumstances in which the courts have held disclosure to be justifiable is the case of *W* v *Egdell* ([1990] 1 All ER 454). Here a patient detained under a restriction order under the Mental Health Act 1983 sought discharge from a mental health review tribunal. His solicitors commissioned a report from an expert, Dr Egdell. Unfortunately for W. this report was unfavourable and the solicitors withdrew the application. Dr Egdell wanted a copy passed to the hospital authorities but the solicitors refused. However, subsequently the report was disclosed to the hospital and was also passed to the Home Office. When W.'s case next came for routine review in front of a Mental Health Review Tribunal the report was adduced. W. brought an action for breach of confidence but failed. In the Court of Appeal it was held that the disclosure was in the public interest. In determining what constituted the public interest they made reference to the GMC guidelines on confidentiality as stated in the Blue Book Professional Conduct and Fitness to Practice. To have failed to have disclosed the information would have meant that information which was relevant to public safety was prevented from reaching the public. The Court of Appeal did however affirm that disclosure could not be made freely available to all and sundry in such a situation and that the information should be disclosed to the appropriate authorities.

One difficult dilemma concerns the GP who is faced with a patient who is HIV positive and refuses to inform his or her sexual partner. In such a situation the doctor should counsel the patient to attempt to facilitate a voluntary disclosure on the patient's part. Nonetheless, should the patient be intransigent the doctor will be faced with the dilemma of whether to disclose despite the patient's opposition. It has been suggested that in such a situation disclosure will be ethically justifiable. The GMC has stated that 'there are grounds for such a disclosure only where there is a serious and identifiable risk to a specific individual who, if not so informed would be exposed to infection' (GMC, 1995). However, this view is not uniformly held. As Lee has argued:

> on each occasion that a confidence is broken in this manner it becomes less likely that at-risk groups will deal with doctors in a sincere basis in the future. As trust is reduced, so too is the capacity of health care professionals to contain the spread of the virus. The promise of professional confidence becomes conditional with the physician reserving the right to waive guarantees previously given. Patients may refuse to deal with health professionals who engage in such confidence tricks.
>
> (Lee, 1994)

Nonetheless, it is suggested that in an extreme situation disclosure to a spouse/identifiable partner is likely to be held to be justifiable were an action for breach of confidence to be brought before the courts.

What of the patient who is epileptic and who the doctor regards as being unfit to drive? In such a situation the patient should be counselled by the GP as to the inadvisability of continuing to drive. But if the patient still maintains that s/he intends to drive and the GP regards this as constituting an unjustifiable risk, then the GMC recommend that the doctor should immediately disclose 'relevant medical information' to the medical advisor at the Driver and Vehicle Licensing Authority (GMC, 1995). The DVLA is the body which has the legal responsibility to determine whether individuals are fit to drive. The GMC also recommend that prior to this disclosure the patient should be informed by the doctor of his/her intention to disclose and that in addition once the DVLA has been informed the doctor should also write to the patient to confirm that disclosure has been made.

THE CHILD PATIENT

Where the patient is a child problematic issues can arise. Where a child is over 16 s/he has a statutory right to consent to medical, surgical and dental treatment (Family Law Reform Act 1969 §8). A child under 16 years of age may be able to consent to treatment if the doctor decides that the child has sufficient maturity to do so (*Gillick* v *West Norfolk and Wisbech AHA* [1985] 3 All ER 402). It is assumed that where a child is over 16 then that child is able to make decisions regarding disclosure of his/her personal information. While it is the case that wherever possible a doctor should respect her patient's wishes, difficult situations may arise. A well-known dilemma concerns the GP faced with a young girl who wants to withhold from her parents the fact that she is seeking contraceptive advice. In such a situation it appears generally accepted that, subject to an assessment that the patient has sufficient maturity to be involved in such treatment decisions, the GP would be justified in withholding the information. What of the young boy with venereal disease. Should this information be disclosed to his parents? The doctor would have to assess the situation and judge the maturity of the particular child before him when reaching that decision. Such decisions can only be made on a case by case basis but such discretion should be exercised with care.

UNAUTHORIZED DISCLOSURE AND SUPPORT STAFF IN SURGERIES

One aspect of some concern is the unauthorized disclosure of patient information. This can happen easily in the context of health care practice. Doctors discuss patients' cases with colleagues. Such discussion should take place in a work environment. Identifiable disclosures of patient information in private situations such as a bar or restaurant are unethical and could result in legal action as well as disciplinary proceedings being brought against the doctor in question.

Maintenance of confidentiality is particularly important, but equally problematic, in the context of a GP's surgery in a small community where the members of that community are well known to the receptionists. The staff of the practice should also have impressed upon them the need to maintain confidentiality, a requirement which should be included in their contract of employment, and that unauthorized disclosure could result in disciplinary proceedings.

The confidentiality of patient records should be ensured. This applies not only to information which is held on computer, but the obligation applies equally to information held on manual files. The receptionist who leaves on the desk a named file with the words 'HIV+' on its cover is breaking the confidentiality of highly sensitive patient information.

DISCLOSURE REQUIRED BY LAW

In certain situations a doctor may be required to disclose information by a particular statutory provision, as in the situation of disclosure of information where a patient has a notifiable disease (Public Health Act 1984 §§10–11). A doctor may be called to give evidence in proceedings in a law court and to disclose information concerning her patient's treatment. She must answer the question in such a situation, there is no 'privilege' for medical information entitling her to refuse to disclose, as exists in other jurisdictions, such as in certain US states (McHale, 1993). Should she fail to do so then she is liable to be found in contempt of court and in an extreme situation is at risk of committal to prison.

A policeman enters the surgery and asks to see a patient's records. Should the GP hand these over? In law the doctor is not obliged to do so and is entitled to maintain the confidentiality of the patient's records. This is because medical records are treated as 'excluded' material under the Police and Criminal Evidence Act 1984. Before the police may obtain such information they must obtain a warrant from a circuit judge sanctioning disclosure of the information in question (§9 and sched 1). Statute also legitimates disclosure of medical information where this is required by a person for the purposes of pursuing litigation (Supreme Court Act 1981 §31). (This provision is of somewhat less importance since the Access to Health Records Act 1990 was passed.) Where the GP is concerned that disclosure of the information may be detrimental to the patient's health the court may order that disclosure instead be made to the patient's advisors rather than directly to the patient (§33 (2)). But while the doctor is generally under no automatic duty to answer police questions regarding her patient, a duty may arise in some situations. For example, if a GP treats a patient who has been involved in a road accident s/he may be required to disclose information which may identify a driver in a road traffic offence (Road Traffic Act 1988 §172).

CONFIDENTIALITY – A DUTY TO DISCLOSE?

Confidentiality may be broken where it is in the public interest to do so. But what if the GP considers disclosure, decides against it but then subsequently a third party is harmed. For instance, the patient threatens to harm certain particular family members, the doctor considers disclosure but decides not to act, and then the patient stabs his cousin. Is the doctor to be held liable in law for this failure to disclose? In other jurisdictions health care professionals have been held to be under obligations, whether under statute or at common law, to make third parties aware of risks which their patients may pose. A celebrated instance is the case of *Tarasoff* v *Regents of the University of California* ([1976] 551 P 2d 334, 131 Cal.R.14). A girl rejected a young man who had fallen in love with her. He subsequently uttered threats to kill her to a psychotherapist. The young man, one Mr Poddar, was taken in by the campus police on the advice of the therapist, but was subsequently released when he was thought to present no danger. He later shot and killed the girl, Miss Tarasoff. Her relatives brought an action claiming negligence on the part of the therapist. The Supreme Court of California held the psychotherapist liable in negligence for failure to take reasonable steps to inform the girl's family of the threats which had been made. While subsequent to *Tarasoff* such an obligation has been recognized in a number of states in the USA, such an obligation has never been recognized in English law. In England the courts are circumspect as to the imposition of such duties upon third parties (*Smith* v *Littlewood* [1987] 1 All ER 710) and it is unlikely that the general practitioner would be held liable for failure to disclose in such a situation.

CONFIDENTIALITY AND THE SICK DOCTOR

An important question of confidentiality concerns the doctor who is sick. On what basis is the doctor required to maintain the confidentiality of her medical information? Are patients ever entitled to know that their own doctor is ill? Doctors as patients are entitled to have the confidentiality of their own health care information maintained. So for example, in *X* v *Y* ([1988] 2 All ER 648) a health authority obtained an injunction to prevent further publication by a newspaper of medical information of two GPs who were HIV +. Yet through their practice they may be in a situation in which they may put others at risk of harm. Take for example, the doctor who is infected with hepatitis B (Wright,1997). The DOH guidelines emphasize that

> It is extremely important that HIV infected health workers receive the same rights of confidentiality as any patient seeking or receiving medical care. Occupational physicians who work within strict guidelines with respect to confidentiality, have a key role in this process.
> (Department of Health, 1993: para 7.2)

Nonetheless there is a balance which needs to be struck here. If a health care professional through his/her ill health is placing others at risk then this may justify steps being taken to reduce this risk, in the public interest, if necessary by informing the employer. If a health care professional is allowed to continue in practice this could lead to patients being placed at risk and in addition to litigation being brought by patients who have developed an illness or have been harmed in some way through a health professional's actions. Litigation in this context may take the form of an action in negligence (Wright, 1997). In some instances there is also the prospect of a prosecution of the doctor. In 1995 a Dr Gaud was prosecuted and convicted of the common law offence of public nuisance when he infected a patient under his care with hepatitis B (Mulholland, 1997).

In addition there are some situations in which the confidentiality of a health care professional may have to be broken in order to trace patients who may have been infected. Instances of this have arisen with regards to health care practitioners who continued to work in high risk specialities having developed HIV/AIDS. Risk of HIV/AIDS transmission is less likely to be a problem in the area of general practice medicine, save where, for instance, the general practitioner has been involved in surgical techniques. Where such public disclosures are made it is important to ensure that they are limited as far as possible to what is absolutely necessary.

What of the situation in which GPs see a colleague deteriorating due to heavy drinking. What should they do? The GP may be putting patients at risk because his drinking impairs his work. There is the prospect in a situation in which a GP ultimately breaks down through ill health that reference may be made to the General Medical Council and this may lead to disciplinary proceedings (Mulcahy and Allsop, 1997). Nonetheless, the doctor's colleagues may hesitate before taking any steps to involve outside bodies, out of understandable loyalty. In such a situation should they decide ultimately to disclose and were a subsequent breach of confidence action to arise it is again likely that the disclosure would be held to be in the public interest.

CONFIDENTIALITY AND DATA PROTECTION

Today patient information in the surgery is frequently held in the form of computer records. While this may facilitate practice, at the same time it has led to concern regarding the security of such patient information. Information held on computer must be registered under the Data Protection Act 1984 (§5). The Data Protection Act 1984 provides that those persons holding data on computer must comply with what are known as the 'Data Protection principles' (Data Protection Act 1984 sched. 1). These require that information must be accurate and that in addition it must be no more detailed than is necessary under the circumstances. Information may only be disclosed to the class of subjects held on the Register. The operation of the Act is overseen by an officer, the Data Protection Registrar, and contravention of the legislation constitutes a criminal offence. A patient whose information has been disclosed without authorization or where there are inaccuracies in the computerized records may claim compensation (§§22 and 23). Information held on manual files has, up to the present, not been subject to the same safeguards, but this is to change. The Data Protection Act 1998 implements the European Union Data Protection Directive (95/46/EC) and when it comes into force it will replace the Data Protection Act 1984. This legislation provides safeguards for data held both on computer and on manual files in 'relevant filing systems' (s1(1)) (Lloyd, 1998). There will be a transitional period for manual data held on relevant filing systems until the Act comes into force.

Patients today have rights of access to their own records whether held on computer or on manual files where this information was created after 1991 (Data Protection Act 1984 and Access to Health Records Act 1990). It should be noted that such rights of access are not absolute and that, for example, information may be withheld where disclosure may endanger the patient's physical or mental health (Data Protection (Subject Access Modification)(Health) Order 1987 SI 1987 No. 1903 as amended). As far as the ownership of these files is concerned, it appears that the view of the Department of Health is that these are owned by the health authority (as successor to the Family Health Services Authority) because they are compiled on forms supplied by the authority (Montgomery, 1997: 251).

GPs frequently are requested to write reports for employers/insurers regarding their patients. This is regulated by the Access to Medical Reports Act 1988. Such reports should not be written without the patient's consent having been obtained by the employer/insurer (s3(1) and section 9). The Act grants the patient the right to see and comment upon the report before it is sent by the GP to the employer/insurer and the employer/insurer must notify the patient of this right. This right may be withheld where the GP is of the view that disclosure is likely to cause serious physical and mental harm to the patient's health or that of others or would indicate a practitioner's intentions towards the patient (§6 (2)).

CONCLUSIONS

As can be seen from the foregoing discussion the present situation presents the general practitioner with many difficult dilemmas. There is much legal uncertainty in this area. Can this position be improved? One option is that of the introduction of legislation regulating the disclosure of health care information. There was an attempt to introduce such legislation in

1995 in the form of a bill drawn up by the British Medical Association in conjunction with bodies representing other health care professionals such as the UKCC, which was placed before parliament in the form of the Disclosure of Health Information Bill 1996. The bill was given a second reading but did not progress further. It contained the basic obligation of confidentiality and then listed a wide range of exceptions to the general principle which were regarded as being justifiable. Again then ultimately much discretion would be left in the hands of the doctor. An alternative proposal, made a number of years ago by the Law Commission to place the common law of breach of confidence upon a statutory footing, whilst facilitating to a certain extent clarification of the law would lead to many of the same problems in ascertaining what is meant by public interest (Law Commission, 1981). It is submitted that some codification and clarification of the law in this area would be desirable. That does not mean, however, that statutory reform would represent a panacea. Whilst law may facilitate medical practice by setting out more clearly the boundaries of disclosure, ultimately it is the doctor him/herself who is left to make such difficult ethical decisions personally.

REFERENCES

Department of Health (1993) 'Protecting health care workers and patients from hepatitis B', *Health Service Guidance* (93)40.

Department of Health (1996) *Protection and Use of Patient Information*, London: DOH.

General Medical Council (1995) *Confidentiality*, London: GMC.

Jones, M. (1990) 'Medical confidentiality and the public interest', *Professional Negligence*, 6: 16.

Law Commission (1981) *Breach of Confidence*, Report No. 110, London: HMSO.

Lee, R.G. (1994) 'Deathly Silence' in R.G. Lee and D. Morgan (eds) *Deathrites* London: Routledge.

Lloyd, I. (1998) *Guide to the Data Protection Act 1998*, London: Butterworth.

McHale, J. and Fox, M. (with J. Murphy) (1997) *Health Care Law: Text and Materials*, London: Sweet & Maxwell, Chapter 8.

McHale, J.V. (1993) *Medical Confidentiality and Legal Privilege*, London: Routledge.

Montgomery, J. (1997) *Health Care Law*, Oxford: Oxford University Press.

Mulcahy, L. and Allsop, J. (1997) *Regulating Medical Work*, Buckingham: Open University Press.

Mulholland, M. (1997) 'Public nuisance: a new use for an old tool', *Professional Negligence*, 11: 70.

Select Committee on the Parliamentary Commissioner (1988–9) Second Report of the Committee on the PCA HC 433.

Warren, E. and Brandise, L. (1890) 'The right to privacy', *Harvard Law Review* 193.
Wright, M. (1997) 'Health care workers and HIV screening', *Journal of Social Welfare and Family Law* 19 (1): 16.

GLOSSARY OF LEGAL TERMS

All ER	All England Law Reports
Cal. R	Californian Law Reports
EU Directive	European Union Directive

Chapter 5

Patient-centredness

A history

Carl May and Nicola Mead

INTRODUCTION

Contemporary medicine is awash with ideas about the *patient-as-person*. Enablement, empowerment, negotiation and patient-centredness all form a vital part of a professional vocabulary that stresses that the role of the doctor is to respond in some new way to the patient as an experiencing individual, rather than as a representative object of organic or psychogenic pathology. In general practice, especially, the patient-as-person is given enormous significance as a partner in the often complex negotiations that take place in the consultation. As, increasingly, the quality of doctor–patient interaction has become a proxy measure for quality of care, patient-centredness is expressed in the construction of formal models of doctor–patient interaction.

While these formal models are a novel innovation in recent medical thinking, what underlies them may not be. In this chapter we will consider the history of the patient-as-person as this has been set out in recent accounts, and then lead on to the way in which these formal models represents a real problem for contemporary medicine.

We begin by discussing two important and influential theses in the current historical sociology of medicine. The first of these, offered by Jewson (1976) and echoed in historical studies (Fissell, 1991), is that the rise of scientific medicine in the nineteenth century led inevitably to the disappearance of the 'sick man' from medical cosmology; and the second, offered by Armstrong (1982), is that the 'person' was rediscovered as a medical problem at the end of the interwar period. In the context of these two theses, the more recent growth of medical ideas about patienthood as a 'biopsychosocial' phenomenon can be seen as an attempt to recapture a lost world of medical practice, as well as a recognition that illness and disease are produced by and experienced in complex ecologies. The chapter then turns to some of the more recent material on 'models' of the consultation and the problems of 'communicating' with the patient.

THE DECLINE OF THE PATIENT?

At the end of the eighteenth century medicine was by its very nature holistic and patient-centred. There could be no other source of medical knowledge about the patient other than her or his own account of symptoms, and this knowledge was primarily acquired through listening to this account (May, 1997), and performing observations of the external appearance of the body. The internal and external mechanisms that drove both disease causation and natural history were, in any case, not understood in any meaningful sense. In practice, this meant that:

> Physical examination was therefore not practised, as it would have served little purpose. Treatment was in any case along general lines and followed a set routine of evacuation, counter-irritation and the administration of 'specifics'. ... Diagnosis was arrived at by what was called an 'estimate of symptoms and appearances'.
>
> (Macalpine and Hunter, 1969: xvi)

In this model of practice, Jewson has noted, there was none of the distinction between psyche and soma that is made by contemporary medicine, and which it finds so troubling (Good, 1994). Instead, these were integral components of the manifestation of illness, equally applicable to the ague (malaria) or habitual temulency (addiction to alcohol). The important thing to note here, was that diagnosis involved a qualitative judgement about the moral state of the patient as much as it did about the appearance of the illness itself; and susceptibility and culpability were intimately linked. In addition, both diagnosis and treatment were negotiable with the patient. In her account of doctors at work in eighteenth-century Bristol, Fissell (1991) describes negotiations about disease causation and treatment that would be familiar to any general practitioner today.

If eighteenth-century medicine was marked by holism and a focus on the subjective and experiential aspects of illness, the nineteenth century was marked by relentless scientific medicalization and somatization, and by the consequent rapid decline in importance of the patient's own account. The shift here was away from *illness* as a subjective (and individualized) experience, towards *disease* as objective (and generalized) phenomena. What mattered in this heroic age of scientific innovation and discovery was the uncovering of discrete and identifiable pathologies. Medicine shifted from the bedside to the hospital, and the medical profession itself became marked by a complex division of labour founded on the emergence of new, scientific specialities. For writers like Jewson, this meant that:

> Interest in the unique qualities of the whole person evaporated to be replaced by studies of specific organic lesions and malfunctions. Disease became a precise and objectively identifiable event occurring within the tissues, of which the patient might be unaware. ... The experiential manifestations of disease, which had previously been the very stuff of illness, were now demoted to the role of secondary signs.
>
> (Jewson, 1976: 235)

Jewson is quite correct, of course, but we must offer a caveat here. The apparent shift from bedside to hospital medicine in the nineteenth century, is of course, followed by a parallel focus in historiography itself. The history of medicine has therefore taken a disproportionate interest in the processes and practices of scientific discovery and the social organization of medicine that were involved in the shift to hospital diagnosis and treatment dominated by the laboratory sciences. The family doctor or general practitioner has thus been marginalized, although we can be confident that such practitioners were still providing the bulk of medical care to the population. If the patient was reduced to the object of medical procedure in the hospital, we have no strong historical evidence that the patient-as-person ceased to matter in family practice.[1] Indeed, the social history (as opposed to the medical history) of general practice remains unwritten in any systematic way.

There is a second reason to be sceptical about Jewson's thesis. For much of the nineteenth century, there was a strong differentiation in the distribution of medical care by social class. The emergent public hospitals – driven as much by the need to locate growing numbers of medical students as by philanthropic motives – primarily catered for the urban working class. The urban elites and the country gentry could be confident of being treated and nursed at home. Because of the highly marked division between Victorian hospital patients (often pauperized and poorly educated) and doctors (often characterized by a rigid middle-class formality), the kinds of interpersonal negotiations that characterized earlier doctor–patient relationships appear far more unlikely. Deference to the doctor can therefore be considered as a function of differential social status, as much as stemming from the subordination of the experiencing subject to the authority of science.

What is absolutely clear is that the patient-as-person vanished from medical textbooks during this period. Physical hygiene and the avoidance of infection became crucial components of the management of the patient, who after all had an increasing probability of being cured, or at least palliated, as a result of the radical growth of medico-scientific knowledge throughout the nineteenth century.[2] This latter point is often neglected by critical histories and sociologies of medicine that focus on the zenith of scientific medicalization (e.g. Arney and Bergen, 1983).

But if the patient-as-person vanished from the medical textbook, as Arney and Bergen suggest, there is not much evidence that the wider medical literature could accommodate such a claim.[3] Victorian medicine grappled with the problem of differentiating between disease as an asocial objective phenomenon to which individuals were susceptible and as a moral problem which arose as the result of individual culpability across a broad range of disease states – from cholera in the 1830s (Morris, 1976) to insanity in the 1880s (Thompson, 1988) – and which often had a hereditarian or eugenicist basis. The important point that needs to be made here is that where the patient-as-person achieves prominence in the medical literature of the late nineteenth century it is primarily as a *moral actor*, that is, in qualitative judgements about the moral character of the patient.

REDISCOVERING THE PATIENT?

The second thesis drawn from historical sociology that we should take note of is advanced by Armstrong (1982). Where Jewson was concerned to show how the patient-as-person disappeared from the medical worldview, and became the passive object of medical knowledge and practice, Armstrong is concerned to show how the patient-as-person was discovered in the interwar period. In particular, he takes as his focus the problems of the 'defaulting' patient and of non-compliance. Once again, this kind of critical literature has initially little to say about the family doctor. What it does demonstrate very effectively is the way in which a new discipline, psychology, was drawn on to redefine the doctor–patient relationship.

Armstrong has shown how the history of ideas about the patient in

British medicine this century has been marked by a shift from seeing the consultation as a meeting in which the patient is the passive recipient of diagnosis and treatment, to one where the patient is considered as a negotiating partner. In part, this has its origins in the influence of ideas about the 'personality' and the 'unconscious' of the patient that took hold in the 1930s (e.g. Brackenbury, 1935). The personality of the patient became one of the key conditions through which non-compliance could be accounted for, and the unconscious was seen as a source of 'blocks' which inhibited recovery. This reflects the growing importance that was attached to broadly psychoanalytic explanations of ill-health at the end of the interwar period (Shorter, 1997).

Central to this new shift was the possibility of negotiation within the consultation, and of the 'problem' of miscommunication between doctor and patient. Concerns about poor compliance had as their corollary a set of ideas that reflected a much stronger relationship between psyche and soma than had been the case at the turn of the century. In part this was derived from wide experience of the physiological effects of psychological trauma during the First World War. But it also reflects a growing sense that community medicine might attend to the patient in a much wider sense. In this context, it is worth noting that medical elites towards the end of the interwar period saw a role for 'social' medicine, which reflected political shifts towards welfarism that had their ultimate and spectacular effect in the Beveridge Report of 1944 and of the creation of the NHS in 1947.

The principal announcement of this much greater range for 'social' medicine may be found in what now seems an unremarkable statement by the secretary of the British Medical Association in 1935:

> the relationship between doctor and patient is not merely between two persons, but between two personalities. ... It is never the body which is out of health, but always the complete being.
>
> (Brackenbury, 1935, cited in Armstrong, 1982)

In retrospect, this is a crucial statement of what we might now characterize as 'holistic' medicine and, importantly, it was aimed primarily at general practitioners. It accomplished two quite distinct ends. First, it suggested that there was no aspect of the patient that could not be, at some level, a problem for which medical attention was not relevant. It thus radically expanded the field of medicine to include the patient's personality and relationships. But second, and for the purposes of this chapter more relevant, it signalled that the doctor was also a potential problem.

The doctor's personality and behaviour might also be a block to achieving the patient's health.

What we have, then, in the period under review, is a shift in the nature of medical judgements about the patient-as-person. Qualitative moral judgements about the patient's character give way to psychological assessments of the patient's personality. The scientific and moral authority of the doctor is similarly displaced by a more problematic professional identity.[4]

THE PATIENT-AS-PERSON IN GENERAL PRACTICE

In general practice the shift to seeing the personality of the patient as being in some way fundamental to the outcome of the consultation reaches its zenith in the work of Michael Balint during the 1940s and 1950s (Balint, 1957). Balint's view was that the 'relationship' between doctor and patient was intrinsically therapeutic and, while the extent to which this influenced doctors in practice is arguable, such a view exercised a considerable influence on general practice's professional elites and especially the embryo Royal College (May *et al.*, 1996). The doctor–patient relationship thus became central to professional doctrine in general practice, in part because it offered a point of departure for a theoretical framework for a kind of medicine that lacked complex diagnostic technologies. It thus offered a means by which general practice could contest the growing threat posed by the rapid growth of hospital medicine in the new National Health Service. This kind of 'model' thus served two distinct purposes: it set up the medical encounter as a therapeutic technique in itself (hence Balint's famous aphorism that *the doctor is the drug*), while at the same time providing a novel means for differentiating general practice from specialized hospital medicine. Where the latter invested its efforts in specific pathological entities, general practice could come to examine the 'whole person' in her or his wider *social* context. This kind of view has gathered increasing momentum: it is the core, for example, of *The Future General Practitioner* (RCGP, 1972) and of much of the educational and exhortative literature that has followed from this (e.g. Neighbour, 1987).

The shift towards 'patient-centred' general practice that is evident throughout the period since 1960 is, of course, much more than a means of securing professional differentiation from hospital medicine. It is also a *moral* enterprise, and this is common to both forms of medicine.

Its clearest exposition may be found in a pivotal statement by a paediatrician:

> The essential unit of medical practice is the occasion when, in the intimacy of the consulting room or sick room, a person who is ill, or believes himself to be ill, seeks the advice of a doctor whom he trusts. This is a consultation and all else in the practice of medicine follows from it.
>
> (Spence, 1960: 271)

The relationship between doctor and patient, therefore, is not simply a technical device for the delivery of medical care, but is founded on bonds of personal obligation and trust. The problem here is that while these may be assumed in the mass of research literature that has emerged since the 1960s, the research-based models of the consultation in general practice that have developed since then have taken as their primary focus the things that doctors *do* with patients, rather than who they *are* to them. That is, they have focused on improving the technical quality of the doctor's activities – by prescribing *style* in the structure, content and duration of the consultation (e.g. Howie *et al.*, 1991). Medical models of the consultation are thus primarily skills based, and treat it as a problem to be resolved through educational interventions.

One way to explain this focus on the consultation as a technical problem of practice is to see medical models of doctor–patient interaction as being propelled by the need to respond to external pressures and wider social trends. Broadly speaking, these have taken the following – intimately connected – forms. First, the period since the 1960s has seen a sustained political critique of medical practice much of which has been derived in part or in whole from the social sciences, in which feminist critiques of patriarchal medical science, and the objectification of the patient, have been especially vocal (Miles, 1991). Second, a slightly later development is the translation of this critique into the advocacy of patient interests through the emergence of ideas about consumerism and their subsequent – but problematic – incorporation into health policy (Fitzpatrick and White, 1997). Finally, there have been structural changes in the organization of primary care resulting from the managerial encirclement of general practice through successive NHS reorganizations (Calnan and Williams, 1995; Dowrick, 1997).

These developments have come together in a way which compounds the doctor as a problem. The 'new' patient-centredness has been ushered in by an extraordinary growth in techniques for modelling the optimum consultation. This is embodied in ideas about 'the patient as expert' (Tuckett *et al.*, 1985), the 'inner consultation' (Neighbour, 1987) and the 'exceptional potential of every consultation' (Stott and Davis, 1979) that reflect both the psychoanalytic antecedents of much of the current literature, and their contemporary reduction to variables in the language and behaviour of the doctor. The purpose of such literature is thus to optimize *technical efficiency* in dealing with the patient.[5] But it also provides a means of setting the doctor's *persona* up as a problem for the patient, hence the emergence of an equally broad literature on patient satisfaction with the consultation, which offers an explicit critique of the doctor in general practice (cf Fitzpatrick and White, 1997).

The problem with this literature is that in pressing the case for the widest possible definition of the patient, it inevitably leads to both resentment about the disparity between 'theory' and 'practice' – which we can observe across the health professions (May, 1992) – and to a practical problem. When the communications skills of general practitioners fail to meet the demands of 'patient-centred' performance indicators, this can only be construed as an individual problem. It is thus a technical deficiency which can perhaps be resolved by training – or reaccreditation.[6] But this literature says rather less about the ways in which structural features of the doctor's work may impinge on the encounter with the patient, or about the more general context in which this takes place. Furthermore, it is often difficult to identify precisely what individual commentators mean by 'patient-centredness', for in theory and practice the definitions employed in the clinical research literature are frequently nebulous. For example, Stewart *et al.* (1995) outline a six component *patient-centred clinical method* which involves:

- exploring both the disease and the illness experience
- understanding the whole person
- finding common ground regarding management
- incorporating health promotion and prevention
- enhancing the doctor–patient relationship
- being realistic

Underpinning this kind of approach to the consultation lies a set of appropriate 'professional attitudes' (Mead, 1997). These include:

- openness to the full range of problems presented by the patient
- interest in and receptiveness to the patient's agenda

- regard for patients as unique individuals with their own beliefs and preferences
- belief in the patient as an expert in his or her own illness
- belief in collaboration and partnership with patients regarding management
- self-awareness of limitations and emotional responses

Stewart *et al.*'s work is but a part of the very extensive literature that attempts to define 'patient centredness' and set out means by which the content and quality of the consultation may be measured in these terms. In the appendix to this chapter, we set out in tabular form some pointers to the way in which this literature has prescribed an appropriate set of 'attitudes' or 'values' for the patient-centred general practitioner. Indeed, patient-centredness is often constructed as a good thing, precisely on moral grounds: it permits the doctor to enter into the patient's own definitions of disease and empowers the patient to speak more openly about her or his problems (McWhinney, 1995; Smith and Hoppe, 1991). It has also been argued that patient-centred consultation styles are more clinically appropriate and effective, since in opening up the consultation they are responsive to patients' perceived needs, and might therefore be expected to lead to improved patient outcomes (i.e. satisfaction, recall, compliance and health outcomes). It may be that such approaches lead to improved outcomes in terms of satisfaction (though even here the evidence is conflicting), but there is much less evidence to suggest that compliance and health outcomes are greatly affected by the doctor's consulting style – partly because many of the measures on which such studies are based have not been properly established as valid or reliable (Mead, 1997). In fact, studies of consulting style have largely shied away from exploring the question of whether there is a demonstrable health gain resulting from patient-centred approaches to the consultation.

The literature on the perfect consultation may therefore isolate the skills of the doctor from the context in which s/he works, and from the objectives of both the doctor and patient. Nor does this model necessarily reinstate the patient as an experiencing individual. Fissell (1991) points to the way in which patients' narratives at the end of the eighteenth century were constructed around proximal cause and long *social* histories. There is no strong evidence that this has changed; indeed current work on the experience of illness suggests precisely the same organization for such accounts (Bury, 1982; Lupton, 1994). There is no place in the five or ten minute consultation for such an expression of subjectivity. Nor, in truth, is there much evidence that doctors want to hear them (Dowrick *et al.*, 1995; May *et al.*, 1996).

CONCLUDING COMMENTS

So how can we account for the expansive nature of 'patient-centredness'? First of all we must emphasize that it represents a moral imperative in contemporary health care: a shift away from the kinds of paternalism that are commonly held to have characterized medicine before the war, and towards seeing health and illness as experiences that *do* impact upon the generality of the patient's well being. In this sense, patient-centredness is about avoiding precisely those facets of the doctor–patient relationship that patients have historically objected to – being treated as a 'disease' rather than a person, not being listened to, not feeling 'cared' for or cared about. Similarly, we can see the growth of patient-centredness as an attempt to empower the patient and to expand their contribution to the consultation. But we should also see patient-centredness – as a way of seeing and acting in the consultation – as part of a wider process in which general practitioners have to work harder to negotiate increasingly complex relationships. Lupton points out that:

> doctors are ... aware that their patients' trust is now no longer necessarily won by virtue of their occupying the role of 'doctor' but must be earned and worked at continually. ... Changes in the medical encounter and the status of doctors are not just a matter of the State, patients or other groups 'gaining' or 'taking' more power from doctors, or vice versa, but involve a series of dynamic and interpersonal negotiations of power centred on the ethic of professional practice.
> (Lupton, 1997: 493)

But it might be that the 'ethic' of patient-centredness, or the values about 'holistic' care that form such a deep and powerful component of professional training for general practice, involve signing up to a series of potent – perhaps irresolvable – problems in the consultation itself. We have sketched out some of the features of the way in which the 'problem' of the patient has changed for medicine over time. Three quite distinct kinds of 'problem' have been identified here: at the zenith of scientific somatization, the patient is a *moral* character; in the shift towards 'social' and ultimately 'biopsychosocial' medicine, the patient is a *psychological* problem; while in the current context – in which patient 'satisfaction' is so prominent a professional and political issue – the patient is increasingly seen as a *critic* of medical practice.

The chapter has focused initially on work that charts the ways in which the patient is lost to, and subsequently rediscovered in, medical discourse. The post-war 'rediscovery' of the patient and the notion that the encounter between doctor and patient is intrinsically therapeutic have, it has been suggested, created a way of seeing the *doctor* as the problem presented by the consultation. The shift here is from the doctor as reflexive listener, striving to make sense of the patient as a person, to the doctor's behaviour as measurable evidence of the deployment of a package of communications skills.

The growth of a literature organized around formal models of patient-centredness (bearing in mind that quality of the consultation is increasingly constituted as a proxy measure for quality of care) has two effects when it is translated into practice. First, it demands ever more of the doctor, perhaps more than we can reasonably expect from a consultation; second, it shifts the focus away from 'relationships' in which the doctor and patient mean something to each other, and are bound together by bonds of trust and obligation, focusing instead on communications 'skills' as a technical achievement.

NOTES

1 Bynum (1994: 29) provides some useful evidence to the contrary.
2 Although there are important debates about whether declining death rates are the result of direct innovation in clinical medicine, or of the extraordinary developments in public health medicine during the nineteenth century, there is no doubt that doctors were much less likely to kill their patients as the result of treatments at the end of the century than they were at the beginning.
3 The real danger here is to assume that the medical textbook corresponds in a direct way to what doctors actually do, when it does not. The purpose of the medical textbook is to outline the things that doctors should *know* about disease before they meet the patient. It is a training manual.
4 It is interesting that it is only once this focus on the psychological aspects of the consultation gets underway that family practice begins to emerge in the literature as a 'space' where the doctor–patient relationship was important.
5 The forms of behaviour that are specified in such approaches simulate those that are to be found in long-standing relationships. One way to understand the growth of ideas about 'patient-centredness' therefore is to see them as a means by which doctors may compensate for the lack of 'in-depth' knowledge about the patient.
6 This is not to say that communications skills are not important, because they

Appendix Professional attitudes associated with patient-centredness (set into the framework proposed by Stewart *et al.*, 1995)

Component (Stewart *et al.*, 1995)	*Examples of professional attitudes / values identified from the literature*
Exploring the disease and illness experience	Openness to full range of patient-presented problems (Stewart *et al.*, 1995); Receptiveness to patients' offers/cues/prompts of expectations, feelings, fears (McWhinney, 1985; Stewart *et al.*, 1995; Grol *et al.*, 1990; Winefield *et al.*, 1996); Openness to 'hidden agenda' (Lipkin *et al.*, 1984); Feels responsible for non-medical aspects of problems (Grol *et al.*, 1990); Positive regard for patients with psychosocial problems, 'non-problems', self-treatable illness, etc. (Cockburn *et al.*, 1987); Interest in behavioural aspects of medicine and speculative thinking (deMonchy, 1992); Sensitivity to what is going on, unconsciously or consciously in the patient's mind (Balint, 1964).
Understanding the whole person	Respects fundamental worth of all patients – belief in value as persons; Respects cultural values of ethnic groups (Stewart *et al.*, 1995); Interest in psychological and social factors in patient's environment (Cockburn *et al.*, 1987); Respect for patient's autonomy, individuality – accepting of diverse backgrounds and personal styles (Lipkin *et al.*, 1984).
Finding common ground regarding management	Willingness to collaborate and share management responsibility with patients (Stewart *et al.*, 1995; Lipkin *et al.*, 1984); Belief in partnership; Openness to patients' differential preferences for decision-making (Cockburn *et al.*, 1987); Willingness to let patients decide on basis of full information; Considers patient basically equal (deMonchy, 1988); Respects patient values, preferences, expressed needs (Delbanco 1992); Regards patient as 'expert' in her or his illness (Tuckett *et al.*, 1985).
Incorporating prevention and health promotion	Enthusiastic interest in three stages of prevention; Willingness to invest time and energy incorporating screening, prevention, health promotion into patient day-to-day care; Values health promotion (Stewart *et al.*, 1995); Values preventive medicine – positive regard for role of GP in preventive care (Cockburn *et al.*, 1987).
Enhancing the patient–doctor	Accepts risks of exposing own weakness and vulnerability, of being hurt; Long-term commitment to patient well-being; Willingness to act as patient advocate (Stewart *et al.*, 1995); Openness to cues of the relationship developing affective relationship (Winefield *et al.*, 1996); Values openness, honesty, information-disclosure; Values for professional role in providing emotional support/counselling (Cockburn *et al.*, 1987); Unconditional positive regard for patients (Lipkin *et al.*, 1984).
Being realistic	Self-awareness of limitations and personal response to stress; Willingness to ask for help when needed (Stewart *et al.*, 1995); Self-awareness of emotional responses (Winefield *et al.*, 1996, Smith and Hoppe, 1991); Considers own opinion as part of team approach (deMonchy, 1992).

so clearly are. The point we emphasize here is that the objective of the general practitioner in the consultation may often be opaque to the expert observer and, more importantly, to the patient.

REFERENCES

Armstrong, D. (1982) 'The doctor–patient relationship: 1930–80', in A. Wright and A. Treacher (eds) *The Problem of Medical Knowledge*, Edinburgh: Edinburgh University Press.

Arney, W. and Bergen, B. (1983) 'The anomaly, the chronic patient and the play of power', *Sociology of Health and illness* 5: 1–24.

Balint, M. (1957) *The Doctor, His Patient and the Illness*, London: Pitman Medical.

Brackenbury, H. (1935) *Patient and Doctor*, London: Hodder and Stoughton.

Bury, M. (1982) 'Chronic illness as biographical disruption', *Sociology of Health and Illness* 4: 167–82.

Bynum, W. (1994) *Science and the Practice of Medicine in the Nineteenth Century*, Cambridge: Cambridge University Press.

Calnan, M. and Williams, S. (1995) 'Challenges to professional autonomy in the United Kingdom: perceptions of general practitioners', *International Journal of Health Services* 25: 219–41.

Cockburn. J., Killer, D., Campbell, E. and Sanson-Fisher, R. (1987) 'Measuring general practitioners' attitudes towards medical care', *Family Practice* 4: 192–9.

Delbanco, T.L. (1992) 'Enriching the doctor–patient relationship by inviting the patient's perspective', *Annals of Internal Medicine* 16: 414–18.

deMonchy, C. (1992) 'Professional attitudes of doctors and medical teaching', *Medical Teacher* 14: 327–31.

deMonchy, C., Richardson, R., Brown, R.A. and Harden, R.M. (1988) 'Measuring attitudes of doctors: the doctor–patient (DP) rating', *Medical Education* 22: 231–9.

Dowrick, C. (1997) 'Rethinking the doctor–patient relationship in general practice', *Health and Social Care in the Community* 5: 11–14.

Dowrick, C., May, C., Richardson, M. and Bundred, P. (1995) 'The biopsychosocial model of general practice: rhetoric or reality', *British Journal of General Practice* 46: 105–7.

Fissell, M. (1991) 'The disappearance of the patient's narrative and the invention of hospital medicine', in R. French and A. Wear (eds) *British Medicine in an Age of Reform*, London: Routledge.

Fitzpatrick, R. and White, D. (1997) 'Public participation in the evaluation of health care',. *Health and Social Care in the Community* 5: 3–8.

Good, B. (1994) *Medicine, Rationality and Experience: An Anthropological Perspective*, Cambridge: Cambridge University Press.

Grol, R., de Maeseneer, J., Whitfield, M. and Mokkink, H. (1990) 'Disease-centred versus patient-centred attitudes: comparison of general practitioners in Belgium, Britain and the Netherlands', *Family Practice* 7: 100–3.

Howie, J., Porter, M., Heaney, D. and Hopton, J. (1991) 'Long to short consultations: a proxy measure of quality for general practice', *British Journal of General Practice* 41, 48–54.

Jewson, N. (1976) 'The disappearance of the sick-man from medical cosmology', 1770–1870', *Sociology*: 10, 225–44.

Lipkin, M., Quill, T.E. and Napodano, J. (1984) 'The medical interview: a core curriculum for residencies in internal medicine', *Annals of Internal Medicine* 100: 277–84.

Lupton, D. (1994) *Medicine as Culture*, London: Sage.

Lupton, D. (1997) 'Doctors on the medical profession', *Sociology of Health and Illness* 19: 480–97.

Macalpine, I. and Hunter, R. (1969) *George III and the Mad Business*, London: Pimlico.

McWhinney, I. (1985) 'Patient-centred and doctor-centred models of clinical decision making', in M. Sheldon, J. Brook and A. Rector (eds) *Decision making in general practice*, London: Stockton.

McWhinney, I.R. (1995) 'Why we need a new clinical method', in M. Stewart, J.B. Brown, W, Weston, I. McWhinney, C. McWilliam and T. Freeman (eds) *Patient-Centred Medicine: Transforming the Clinical Method*, Thousand Oaks: Sage.

May, C. (1992) 'Individual care? Power and subjectivity in therapeutic relationships', *Sociology* 26: 589–602.

May, C. (1997) 'Habitual drunkards and the invention of alcoholism: susceptibility and culpability in nineteenth century medicine', *Addiction Research* 5: 169–87.

May, C., Dowrick, C. and Richardson, M. (1996) 'The confidential patient: the social construction of therapeutic relationships in general practice', *Sociological Review* 44: 187–203.

Mead, N. (1997) *Patient-centredness in the Consultation: Theory and Measurement*, Manchester: National Primary Care Research and Development Centre.

Miles, A. (1991) *Women, Health and Medicine*, Buckingham: Open University Press.

Morris, R. (1976) *Cholera 1832*, New York: Holmes & Meirs.

Neighbour, R. (1987) *The Inner Consultation*, London: Kluwer.

Royal College of General Practitioners (1972) *The Future General Practitioner*, London: RCGP.

Shorter, E. (1997) *The History of Psychiatry: From the Era of the Asylum to the Age of Prozac*, London: Yale University Press.

Smith, R.C. and Hoppe, R.B. (1991) 'The patient's story: integrating the patient- and physician-centered approaches to interviewing', *Annals of Internal Medicine* 115: 470–7.

Spence, J. (1960) 'The need for understanding the individual as part of the training and function of doctors and nurses', in The Purpose and Practice of Medicine, Oxford: Oxford University Press.

Stewart, M., Brown, J., Weston, W., McWhinney, I., McWilliam, C. and Freeman, T. (1995) *Patient-centred Medicine: Transforming the Clinical Method* Thousand Oaks: Sage.

Stott, N. and Davis, R. (1979) 'The exceptional potential in every primary care consultation', *Journal of the Royal College of General Practitioners*, 29: 201–5.

Thompson, M. (1988) 'The wages of sin: the problem of alcoholism and general paralysis in nineteenth century Edinburgh', in W. Bynum, R. Porter and M. Shepherd (eds) *The Anatomy of Madness: Essays in the History of Psychiatry*, London: Routledge.

Tuckett, D., Boulton, M., Olson, C. and Williams, A. (1985) *Meetings between Experts: An Approach to Sharing Ideas in Medical Consultations*, London: Tavistock.

Winefield, H., Murrell, T., Clifford, J. and Farmer, E. (1996) 'The search for reliable and valid measures of patient-centredness', *Psychology and Health* 11: 811–24.

Chapter 6

Ethics and postmodernity

Sam Smith

> We are not moral thanks to society (we are only ethical or law abiding thanks to it); we live in society, we *are* society, thanks to being moral. At the heart of sociality is the loneliness of the moral person. Before society, its law-makers and its philosophers come down to spelling out its ethical principles, there are beings who have been moral without the constraint (or is it luxury?) of codified goodness.
>
> (Zygmunt Bauman, 1993: 61)

Postmodernism, at first glance a suspiciously paradoxical term, is more often associated with art and architecture, literature and literary criticism, than the problems of ethical medical practice. Issues raised by a postmodern perspective may seem far removed from the question of what it is we ought to do, how we should be, when faced in our surgeries, or at a bedside, with the demands, fears, hopes, expectations and choices of our patients. And yet the very legitimacy of questions posed in these now familiar terms, of hopes and fears, demands and expectations, and pre-eminently choices – birthright of Enlightenment emancipation – itself presages a movement away from the modern; away from authority and law, order and certainty, towards a 'meeting of experts' (Tuckett *et al.*, 1985), a diversity of views, lay and medical, each seeking respect and, perhaps in still unequal voices, claiming entitlement. The patient's problem is no longer to be defined and purified by the medical eye which 'grasps the universal' and 'knows the reason why a particular form of healing meets with success' (Gadamer, 1996: 31–2). The problem has become elusive, multifaceted, to be negotiated both in terms of its comprehension and its attempted resolution, and in a manner which even the broadly inclusive triple diagnosis – physical, psychological and social – fails any longer to specify adequately.

Postmodernism, depending upon whose opinion is sought, is alternately challenging, fascinating, irritating, irrelevant, emancipating and for some – the post-postmodern – even *passé*. Postmodernity, if such exists, is the condition embracing postmodernism, the epoch of the postmodern. There are those, for example Anthony Giddens (1991) and Jurgen Habermas (Bernstein, 1985), who would deny postmodernity an epochal status, not recognizing a discontinuous, separate condition, but theorizing in different ways the events, processes and problems of the contemporary social world as a crisis of high modernity. David Harvey, author of the detailed and accessible *The Condition of Postmodernity*, whilst allowing that there may be distinctive characteristics of a postmodern world, theorizes them in terms of the vicissitudes of late capitalism (Harvey, 1990). But reject it or embrace it, like Barry Smart, many insist that postmodernity cannot be ignored, and its characteristic insights and attitudes, whilst contestable, may be here to stay (Smart 1993). Recent articles in both the *British Medical Journal* and the *British Journal of General Practice* suggest that postmodern thinking is beginning to interest and even assume importance for at least some engaging with contemporary medical practice (Hodgkin, 1996; Mathers and Rowland, 1997).

As for myself, I am firmly in the camp of those who find postmodern ideas both fascinating and challenging. And perhaps as a GP this is not so surprising. After all, in each consultation the authority of medical knowledge is likely to be challenged, if only implicitly. We are charged with the task of negotiating understandings, of persuading, empowering, supporting and enabling, rather than legislating and controlling. In this sense we must be open to the other, to the people who, as our patients, grapple to master the threat to selfhood that illness, disease, trauma and even common anxiety represent. And we are obliged to deal with them ethically. But what is it to act ethically, in a postmodern age? At a time when alternatives abound and choice is paramount, when plural values compete and authority is up for grabs, and when uncertainty is the order of the day, are there any substantial and durable principles on which to found an ethics of practice? The question that postmodernity poses for ethical practice is this. Is it possible to develop an ethical code that is anything other than relative to and contingent on the circumstances of the moment? I will return to this question later, but before that, I would like to present a recent encounter with a patient which will serve as a context for further discussion.

This story concerns a woman of 50 who I had seen only infrequently when dealing with routine and hitherto non-serious matters of health. I did not know her well, but our exchanges had felt comfortable enough. It had been some time since her last attendance when, at a routine appointment, she described her experience over the few months previously of a persistent pain in the right side of her chest, worse on taking a deep breath, and when she laughed or coughed. She had lost a few pounds in weight and had felt recently less energetic than usual. She was, however, sleeping and eating well, and continuing to cope with a busy life. She attributed her pain to a muscle strain. She appeared healthy and when I examined her I could find nothing abnormal. Concerned about the persistence of her pain, the weight loss and tiredness, and also because I knew she was a smoker, I suggested a chest x-ray. She said firmly that she did not want to expose herself to x-rays, that she did not want painkillers, but would like me to refer her for homeopathic treatment.

The ethical questions posed by this case, although not dramatic, are manifold and familiar, and I have yet to resolve them. Such questions lead to the twists and turns of moral philosophy and in this chapter, it is to a postmodern moral philosophy that we must look for some sort of answer. It might seem that postmodernism, which often stands accused of relativism, or flirting with a radical scepticism amounting to nihilism, is the last place to seek moral guidance. Postmodern thinking, however, perhaps in response to this criticism, has of latter years taken an ethical turn (Dews, 1995: 6). The works of Zygmunt Bauman and Emmanuel Levinas stand out in their commitment to exploring the possibilities for ethical relationships with others, and I will turn to the ethical philosophy of Levinas later. But first, to highlight the issues involved in arriving at a postmodern ethics, an ethics without foundations, I will outline those features of postmodern thinking which to me seem to question our Enlightenment inheritance so severely.

Postmodernity is most often delineated in opposition to modernity, that period in the development of the western world extending over the past 300 or 400 years since the late Renaissance and eighteenth-century Enlightenment, to some point in the latter half of this century. Although not undisputed, the characteristics of modernity, socio-political, economic, cultural and philosophical, are generally taken to include:

- the growth of secular authority manifest in the development of the nation state;
- the belief that reason and the explanatory accounts of natural science provide a secure foundation for knowledge;
- a belief that man, via an enlightened hegemony, can order his own destiny through rationally determined and implemented projects of economic, technological and social engineering;

- the promulgation of these ideas by, for example, *les Philosophes* as emancipation from tradition, superstition, prejudice and the power of the church;
- the growth of capitalism, industrialization, urbanization and technology;
- the emergence of unifying and universal explanatory theories in natural and human sciences, for example, Newtonian mechanics, Darwinian evolution via natural selection, Marxism, Parsonian structural functionalism and other structuralist theories and biomedical explanations for the causes and treatment of disease;
- the idea of the self as a unitary, self-determining, autonomous agent, transparent to reflexive introspection;
- and a belief in the possibility of a rationally determinable and universally applicable system of morals.

The underlying assumption of modernity is that certain knowledge of the world, ourselves included, is not only possible, but will provide the basis for the ineluctable progress of mankind. Whilst this assumption may now be held a little more tentatively, there is still a common belief that our knowledge of the world, particularly as scientifically established, will more and more closely approximate reality, that is, the truth (Weinberg, 1993: 132–51). Providing foundations for certainty was a task philosophy set itself. The conflicting conclusions of the Ancients, on the one hand the universal, transcendent truth of Plato's ideas, on the other the particular, observable and demonstrable truths of Aristotle, were reworked via Cartesian rationalism, founded on the clear and certain ideas of the centred subject, and the empiricism of Hume and Locke which 'could only expect success, by following the experimental method, and deducing general maxims from a comparison of particular instances' (Hume, 1975: 174). Hugh Silverman suggests it was Kant's attempted resolution, bringing together 'a rational subject as a transcendental unity of apperception with the manifold of experience', and claiming that the 'metaphysical foundations of all experience would rest in the transcendental domain of pure reason' (Silverman, 1993: 4), which held sway, albeit not without dispute, until the end of the nineteenth century.

By that time the assumptions of modernity were under threat, not only philosophically, notably at the hands of Friedrich Nietzsche, but also because the increasingly manifest human cost of industrialization and urbanization was calling unbridled progress, at least of a capitalist variety, into question. In the next fifty years, two world wars would so tarnish the ideal of progress as to cast doubt deep into the heart of mankind. It was not that modernity's progressive, rational ideal had not always had its critics. John Keats lamented Newton's prismatic 'unweaving of a rainbow' and Max Weber foresaw the disenchantment of the world imprisoned in an iron cage of bureaucratic rationalization. But doubt is mother to anxiety and provokes either a restless search for alternative foundations, or a more radical mistrust unleashing a reckless urge to do without foundations altogether. It is in this sense that the hallmark of postmodernity is seen by Zygmunt Bauman, one of the foremost commentators on postmodernity, as a crisis of legitimation (Bauman, 1992). Jean-François Lyotard, whose report on the state of knowledge in the western world is sometimes seen as having ushered in postmodernity, agrees that within contemporary society and culture, in contrast to the Enlightenment, 'the question of the legitimation of knowledge is formulated in different terms. The grand narrative has lost its credibility' (Lyotard, 1984).

If this incredulity is, as Lyotard suggests, a characteristic of postmodernity, then there are many reasons for it. Perhaps foremost among them is the apparent collapse of the dichotomized progressivist ideal due, in the West, to the threat to local, national and global well-being of unrestrained capitalism and its apparently double-edged technology, and in the East to the demise of Soviet Marxism. The institutionalized reflexivity of modern society renders social and scientific systems susceptible to chronic revision in the light of new information, knowledge and attitudes (Giddens, 1991). Science itself, bastion of Enlightenment certainty, by this very fact becomes uncertain, its truth provisional, and as Thomas Kuhn (1970), for instance, has argued, is far from the progressively cumulative enterprise it was considered to be.

The explosive advance in information and communications technology not only intensifies such reflexive processes, but undermines credulity in other ways. The IT revolution has the effect of compressing time and space (Harvey, 1990), thereby contributing to what Anthony Giddens terms disembedding mechanisms, which 'separate [human] interaction from the particularities of locales' (Giddens, 1991: 20). If people of the developed world may now be said to inhabit a global village, it is one without the reassuring habits, customs and communal worldview of traditional village life, bound by place and time. Furthermore, instant media analysis, or manipulation, is now capable of undermining the most authoritative of voices. Indeed, so convincing are the simulacra of contemporary commodity and image production that some, for example Jean Baudrillard, say there is no longer a meaningful difference between the real and the simulated (Baudrillard, 1988). The stakes are high and risk is a fact of daily life; on one hand the opportunity of boundless possibility and on the other catastrophe.

Philosophically, it was pre-eminently Nietzsche who called into question the universalizing pretensions of the Enlightenment project. He pointed out that the construction of knowledge was inevitably perspectival and historical and as such always relative; reality, in a sense, a fiction. More dramatically, he proclaimed the 'death of God', thereby implying the end of certainty, at least as founded in any transcendent realm (Smith, 1996: 71). All claims to such truth, Nietzsche believed, could be unmasked to reveal the ultimate and absolute reality, the will-to-power (Lyon, 1994: 8). Although reacting to what he saw as the nihilism of an anaemic Christian morality, to many, such irrationalism, when 'reason's doubt turns on reason itself', likewise forebodes nihilism . Understandably Nietzsche's conclusions have been resisted, but other philosophers have continued the work of dismantling modernity's pretensions in different ways.

Whilst there is little explicit about ethics or morality in Wittgenstein's work (Hekman, 1995), the conclusions of his later writings – that there could be no such thing as a private language and that ultimately meaning, and truth, depend on 'forms of life' – also point towards relativism. The crucial role that language plays in determining truth, recognized by Wittgenstein and others, precipitated the so-called 'linguistic turn' in philosophy. On the continent, the new attention to language was largely inspired by Ferdinand de Saussure's structural theory of linguistics. One of the axioms of Saussure's system is the arbitrary nature of the sign. According to Saussure there is no absolutely determined or determinable connection between a word, the signifier or sign, and signified, the object in reality to which it refers. Some recent continental thinkers have exploited this axiom in pursuit of anti-foundationalist aims (Norris, 1996: 43–6).

Taken to its extreme in post-structuralist thought, for example in that of Derrida, 'reality' *is* the signifier, at least in so far as what we 'know' of reality we can only know through language. And language, the system of signifiers, assumes its meaning, not from the immutable reference of words, but as a text. Meaning inheres ambiguously in the signifying chain and is, hence, open to interpretation. Consequently no single interpretation can claim, over any other, to be the truth. For Michel Foucault, one of the most influential of contemporary thinkers, this means that 'reality and truth are wholly linguistic or discursive constructs' (Norris, 1996: 9) which, furthermore, are constituted by relationships of power within discourse. The world, including ourselves as subjects, becomes unknowable except in terms of a discourse which itself sets the limits of meaningful debate. In similar vein, Richard Rorty maintains that truth is a matter of 'final vocabularies' rather than absolutely given (Rorty, 1989).

The thrust of such anti-foundationalist, historicized philosophy, therefore, is to 'finally dispense with all notions of "truth" save that which treats it (in Nietzschean fashion) as a product of the epistemic will-to-power' (Norris, 1996: 9). This leaves the concept of a moral agent in a rather precarious position if, in a sense, he or she is a spoken rather than a speaking subject, and can make no appeal to any objective, universal and abiding truth.

The sustained postmodern assault on modern conceptions of truth and certainty seems for many to threaten chaos, amoral relativism or nihilism; a culture where anything goes and which substitutes aesthetics for ethics, leaving a personally felt anxiety about meaning and selfhood. To others it signifies emancipation, jouissance and the freedom of aesthetic self-realization. There are some, for example Umberto Eco, who see parallels with other troubled times, such as the end of the first millennium in Europe (Smart, 1993: 29). Indeed, postmodern scepticism may itself be just the current expression of doubt, culturally endemic at least in post-traditional times. To quote Anthony Giddens, 'the integral relation between modernity and radical doubt is an issue which, once exposed to view, is not only disturbing to philosophers but is *existentially troubling* for ordinary individuals' (1991: 21). Lyotard (1984: 77) puts it somewhat more elliptically when he states that 'Modernity, in whatever age it appears, cannot exist without a shattering of belief and without the discovery of the "lack of reality" of reality, together with the invention of other realities'. The postmodern, to be truly postmodern, would seem, paradoxically, to have to attempt a position which excludes the possibility of this closure.

In contrast, the Enlightenment project, following the successes of the natural sciences, had set the human sciences the task of discovering universal laws governing social processes. The enlightened aspiration was that such knowledge would enhance systems of social organization and political control. But as Barry Smart says, 'It is no longer possible to attach any credence to the idea of secure epistemological foundations, or the notion of political guarantees' (1993: 80). Because of its reflexively self-constituting nature, society is inherently unpredictable. If so, we would seem to be faced with having to abandon the hope of a collective, legislative moral politics based on a secure understanding of social processes. Furthermore, we may have to abandon a subject-centred morality, if the subject is but a discursive construct whose morality is contingent on a relative and historically situated discourse, and is thereby denied appeal to (non-existent) universal moral truths. In such an uncertain world, however, the question of moral agency, individual or social, seems to gain greater urgency.

There are many responses to this problem, liberal, communitarian, feminist and neo-Marxist, postmodern or otherwise, which seek to address the issue of collective and individual morality, and favour differing concepts of subjectivity and society. The concept of morality is inseparable from the concept of subjectivity. Morality does not exist without moral choices or moral acts and the moral agents responsible for them. What sort of morality is possible, therefore, depends on what sort of subject we are dealing with. Whether the subject is an autonomous self or a discursive self, free or determined, rational or expressive, intellectual or embodied, whole or divided, has been and continues to be a matter of debate.

The 'authorized version' of the secret of selfhood, Roy Porter contends, is 'commonly seen to lie in authenticity and individuality, and its history is presented as a biography of progress towards that goal, overcoming great obstacles in the process' (Porter, 1997: 1). But it might be argued that this view of the self lies at the intersection of at least three separate discourses: autonomously and progressively modern, a dash of Romantic heroism, and an implicitly psychologistic undertone of maturational development. If, as some would maintain, discourse dictates the conditions of possible understanding, then the rug is effectively pulled from under such an aspiring self's feet. The problem seems to be to try and square the sense of ourselves as free, self-determining, embodied, perceiving agents, the loci of our thoughts and personal knowledge, authors of our own actions, with the realization that we are acted on by the 'world out there', or by the 'inner world', by other people, by forces greater than ourselves that motivate, inhibit, constrain or liberate, in a way that is often, alarmingly, not only beyond our control, but beyond our understanding. It would seem that the resulting messiness of experience is sufficiently unpredictable, and the enigma of the world sufficiently impenetrable, to elude the rational grasp of the grand, explanatory narratives of modernity.

Where does this leave us in our attempts to respond ethically to our patients, and what of those questions I was pondering earlier concerning my own patient? Or is medicine 'curiously immune to these epidemic uncertainties', as Paul Hodgkin (1996) maintains? As doctors, and possibly as patients too, we may agree with him when he says:

> Health is one of the few remaining social values that garners unambiguous support. This is largely due to our continuing and

> communal belief that there is one truth 'out there' which can be known, understood, and controlled by anyone who is rational and competent.
>
> (Hodgkin, 1996: 1568)

How, indeed, can we act ethically, as doctors, if we do *not* subscribe to this view? We can be kind, sympathetic, even empathic, accommodating, sensitive, and yet in the end, as doctors, do we not have to act in accordance with our *medical* beliefs? Or should we, because we no longer trust the promise of evidence-based medicine, or no longer wish to assert our power within the medical discourse, modify these beliefs, make them provisional, no better, in fact, than any other belief? With respect to my patient above, does homeopathy, even though I do not understand how it can possibly work, offer the prospect of as much benefit as orthodox medicine? Or does the fact of her inclination and choice obviate such a question in a postmodern world? The problem is not so much whether it is ethical to advise her of my point of view, to present the facts and possibilities as I understand them, and let her choose, or how assiduously I should attempt to persuade her towards my favoured course of action. It is more to do with how I come to have an ethical point of view at all. In the words of Zygmunt Bauman:

> The ethical paradox of the postmodern condition is that it restores to agents the fullness of moral choice and responsibility while simultaneously depriving them of the comfort of the universal guidance that modern self-confidence once promised.
>
> (Bauman, 1992: xxii)

If we accept the postmodern diagnosis it would seem that we are left facing the task of constructing an ethics without foundations from a self without foundations.

A first step might be to accept that whilst uncertainty appears to be a condition of our self constitution, morality is also: to be a self of whatever sort is to be a moral self. This is not to claim that humans, although endowed with a moral sense, have within them some distillable and universal Good, perhaps some sort of telos to which they inevitably aspire. Who could hope to define such a good? Nor is it to claim that there are moral laws uniquely derivable by effort of human reason, in a Kantian or Rawlsian fashion, which ensure that Good will accompany their enactment. Nor yet is it to suggest, as Richard Rorty might, that our moral beliefs are merely contingent and that we can abstract ourselves from them and examine them at will (Hekman, 1995: 157). Rather it is to suggest that we inevitably, necessarily rather than contingently, hold beliefs about what is right and wrong. As Susan Hekman says 'morality is constitutive of subjectivity: my moral beliefs make me who I am' (1995: 157). And, we might add, to hold a belief is to believe that it is true prior to any thought of justification. A belief, including a moral belief, does not require justification unless or until it is called into question.

What, then, calls into question our moral beliefs? Susan Hekman (1995), adopting a broadly Foucauldian and feminist orientation, develops an account of a discursive self and hence a discursive morality. Selves and morality are together constituted in what she calls, following Wittgenstein, the 'language games' of human discourse. Moral beliefs are contested within moral discourse. Discourse for Foucault, however, involves power and the subjection of the subject. But the subject is saved from being fully determined or 'spoken' by the dominant discourse in two respects. First, discourse is inevitably ambiguous and endlessly capable of reinterpretation, and second power 'produces not only domination, but resistance to domination – freedom' (Hekman, 1995: 83). Taken together this means not only that the subject has room for creative self-construction, but also, '*because* we cannot assume that subjectivity is a given, therefore we must take moral responsibility for the construction of ourselves as subjects'. With regards to my patient above, her choice of homeopathy may in some ways represent resistance to the discourse of biomedicine, which seems to offer so much and yet threatens so much at the same time. Her choice as an expression of resistance, rather than, say, a choice between, apples and pears, or a Ford or a Vauxhall, appears to be an ethical one.

I think there are problems with a discursive approach to the self and morality. First when it is claimed that we are morally responsible for the construction of ourselves as subjects, I am left wondering who, exactly, is 'we'. Are we not left having to answer the question of subjectivity all over again? Second, choice as resistance may have an ethical appeal, but if it is so, how do we differentiate, in terms of ethical value, between self-constructive choices, say, to be a Ford owner as opposed to a Vauxhall owner, or to die according to an advance directive? Does not this indeed collapse ethics into aesthetics? Furthermore, it is not quite clear how even a discursively self-constructed subject becomes socially responsible except by having the limits of his or her individual morality constrained by a communal moral discourse. In which case to what extent is that self-constructive? We would seem to be trapped within an endlessly iterative process of power and resistance, constraint and emancipation, becoming and dissolution, called forth and cast down alike by the very same discourse, which refuses to shoulder the burden of any definitive truth. To aspire to anything more is hopelessly modern.

Modernity proclaimed the power of reason, the hope of certainty and faith in progress. If it has been superseded by postmodernity, lauding diversity, relativity and choice, it is not as a further stride in the march of history but, with progress bereft of meaning, as the end of history. In a postmodern world difference becomes pivotal. Plurality, diversity, choice – all entail difference. Indeed, for many, it is the positive affirmation of difference, of the other, that confers on postmodernity its emancipatory potential and extends a rescuing hand to morality. Plural discourse at least renders possible the interruption of different voices – ethnic, feminist, poor and oppressed, patient and consumer; a space for the voice of the other, albeit a space in which no voice, perhaps, can claim a superiority immune to deconstructive unmasking.

In the postmodern search for morality the other, or Other, takes centre stage. The relation with the Other is the primordial ethical relation; it is within the relation of I to Other that the foundation of morality, however fragile and elusive, may be apprehended. Of recent moral philosophers, Emmanuel Levinas is thought by many to have explored this relation with greatest insight and subtlety, and it is to his ethical philosophy, in so far as I understand it, that I would like to turn before concluding.

There is no space in a chapter such as this to give an account of the evolution of Levinas' thought or to do justice, were I able, to its depth and complexity. He is held largely responsible for introducing the phenomenology of Husserl and Heidegger to French philosophy, although his mature work has outgrown – even abandoned – its origins. First published in 1961, *Totality and Infinity* is perhaps his major philosophical work, but he has also written extensively on religion and the Talmud, in many ways pursuing the same moral themes (Davis, 1997).

Above all else, and key to his philosophy, is Levinas' insistence on the radical alterity of the Other. As such, the Other is not simply another person, much like myself, understood in my own terms, captive of the ego. The Other is a concept beyond adequation; like infinity, it overflows any conceptualization and is uncontainable within any totality.[1] The Other thereby stands outside any universalizing theory, which would inevitably entail a 'reduction of the Other to the Same' – a reduction of the Other to another being or existent within an ontology of Being (Levinas, 1969: 43).

The Other is not, therefore, objectifiable in a scientific sense. Total alterity, Levinas says, 'does not shine forth in the *form* by which things are given to us, for beneath form things conceal themselves' (1969: 192).

Whatever science may tell us of relations, the scientific penetration of objects reveals only new forms and further surfaces – perhaps ultimately the unimaginable, mathematical surfaces of superstrings – behind which, in Kantian obscurity, things-in-themselves remain hidden. Thus concealed, only to be glimpsed, the Other provokes an insistent but unrequitable desire, which scientific understanding does not satisfy. As Levinas says 'the metaphysical desire tends toward *something else entirely*, toward the *absolutely other*' (1969: 33).

How, then, can such an opaque and inconceivable Other have any impact upon us or our morality? Although difficult to express, the answer seems to me to have a compelling logic. If the Other's otherness is taken as absolute, any relation with the Other must demand as its second term an absolute identity; only thus can the two terms of the relation remain inviolate. In my relation to the Other my identity must be absolute (no part of it 'other', for instance a construct of discourse), and the Other must be absolutely other; neither term capable of incorporating or being incorporated. In the context of such a relation, therefore, my identity, my subjectivity, must constitute an 'I' prior to any ontology or any discursively constructed self. As Levinas says, whatever happens to me, whatever I am thinking, whatever I might think myself to be, the '"I" is identical in its very alterations' (1969: 36). To my mind, this seems to answer to a phenomenological truth about myself. But most importantly, whilst granting my identity, this relation to the Other at the same time rescues me from being 'enchained' by my identity; it provides an exit from solipsism.

A second and crucial consequence of the inviolability of its terms is that the relation to the Other is asymmetrical, or non-reciprocal. As Levinas maintains, it is not a simple, reversible correlation: 'The reversibility of a relation where the terms are read indifferently from left to right and from right to left would couple them *one* to the *other*; they would complete one another in a system visible from the outside' (1969: 35). If such were the case the transcendence of the Other would be violated. It is this irreversibility, this lack of reciprocity, that confers on the relation with the Other its ethical nature, and I will return to this shortly. Furthermore, because the relation of I and Other cannot become a 'we', moral responsibility in my relation to the Other is mine alone.

The non-reciprocity of the I/Other relation means that it cannot be a being-with, and here Levinas departs from the philosophy of his early teacher, Martin Heidegger. Morality, at its source, springs from my desire of the Other, a reaching out towards the not-me. If the primary relation with others were between beings-in-the-world – that is, being-with or

Mitsein, embraced within the totality of Being – otherness and identity would be compromised, and there would be no spark to the moral impulse. As Levinas says, this would 'subordinate the relation with *someone*, who is an existent, (the ethical relation) to a relation with the *Being of existents*, which … subordinates justice to freedom'. He continues, 'In subordinating every relation with existents to the relation with Being the Heideggarian ontology affirms the primacy of freedom over ethics' (1969: 45). As equal beings we may claim or even grant each other freedom, but freedom itself is not ethical. It entails no obligation to the other, unless by fiat, and we may agree with Zygmunt Bauman when he asserts that morality must precede 'codified goodness'.

Non-reciprocity entails a relation of being-for rather than being-with. I cannot expect that the Other will treat me as I treat him. The moral burden of my actions is, therefore, entirely mine. There is no hiding place within moral law, nor comfort in the hope of reciprocal consideration. Bauman neatly captures this irreversibility in the following juxtaposition: '"I am ready to die for the Other" is a moral statement; "He should be ready to die for me" is, blatantly, not' (Bauman, 1993: 51).

According to Levinas, the Other appears to me as a face. The primary ethical relation is face to face; a relation of two inviolate terms. There can be no third term linking them within a totality. But the face is not the ordinary, sensible face of my experience, the face of another like me, but rather the epiphany of the Other. As such it is always mysterious. In the presence of the face I am drawn into speech, as if hoping to forge a link, to bridge the abyss between us. Discourse is child to this urge to speak. To quote Levinas:

> The relation between the Other and me, which dawns forth in his expression, issues neither in number nor in concept. The other remains infinitely transcendent, infinitely foreign; his face in which his epiphany is produced and which appeals to me breaks with the world that can be common to us, whose virtualities are inscribed in our *nature* and developed by our existence. Speech proceeds from absolute difference.
>
> (Levinas, 1969: 194)

But it is only in *saying* that the moral impulse is given breath. Once said, discourse falls prey to deconstruction and, as we have seen, morality, codified or otherwise, becomes the victim. To be wholly discursive constructs, as Hekman might aver, selves would have to surrender their inviolate status, and the possibility of an ethical relation, if the arguments outlined above are accepted, would be surrendered. Once violated, we are no longer selves.

I would like to conclude this chapter by briefly exploring the relevance of this ethical philosophy for the case of my patient, but there remains a final step to be taken. As I have indicated, the ethical relation with the Other, from which my morality springs, cannot be pluralized. Expressed thus, however, it is an abstraction. My relation to the Other does not refer to a particular meeting with another person in historical time. And yet, obviously, there are other people in the world who exist and with whom I interact. The Other is only ever an epiphany or revelation; a reality, albeit an inexpressible reality, whose face appears at moments of desire, of awe or mystery, or is forced upon my attention as trauma. The Other, calling me into existence and rupturing my solitude, makes me aware of the possibility of others, and awakens me to the fact that to my neighbour, I am other. Whilst leading me out of solitude into society, this does not absolve my personal moral responsibility nor render this morality expressible in universal terms. Nevertheless, at least it allows me hope of being treated morally, albeit not reciprocally, in so far as I am Other for others.

When faced by my patient in the consulting room I am morally responsible for her as Other. Likewise, she too is responsible for me although she may not be aware of this. My moral obligation, however, cannot depend on hers, whether or not she is aware of it. Morally, I cannot impose on her the weight of my medical proscription, however well-founded on evidence. To do so would be to violate her. On the other hand, her request may not be made in the light of any real respect for me and my otherness as doctor. Indeed, she may not understand this, just I may not understand her. How then should we proceed? Face to face we are each in the presence of the Other. In so far as we are able to maintain this relation we act morally towards one another. We can only speak out and negotiate the possibilities.

It seems apt, in support of this conclusion, to finish this chapter as I started, by quoting Zygmunt Bauman:

> Negotiation implies an ongoing process, but also a process without a direction guaranteed before hand, nor one whose outcomes can be securely anticipated. In such a setting, the triumph of morality is in no way assured in advance; it is touch and go all the way. Neither solemn preaching nor stern legal rules will do much to make the fate of morality less precarious. It is the realisation that this is the case, that all and any promises to stop this being the case are – must be – naive or fraudulent, that is morality's best chance. It is also its only hope.
>
> (Bauman, 1993: 183)

NOTE

1 To my mind, the Other cannot thereby be the source or origin or container of anything and, hence, is unlike any usual conception of God. Levinas does, however, seem to make this equation when discussing and elaborating Descartes' ontological proof (1969: 211).

REFERENCES

Baudrillard, J. (1988) *America*, London: Verso.

Bauman, Z. (1992) *Intimations of Postmodernity*, London: Routledge.

—— (1993) *Postmodern Ethics*, Oxford: Blackwell.

Bernstein, R. (1985) *Habermas and Modernity*, Cambridge: Polity Press.

Davis, C. (1997) *Levinas: An Introduction*, Cambridge: Polity Press.

Dews, P. (1995) *The Limits of Disenchantment*, London: Verso.

Gadamer, H-G. (1996) *The Enigma of Health*, Cambridge: Polity Press.

Giddens, A. (1991) *Modernity and Self-Identity*, Cambridge: Polity Press.

Harvey, D. (1990) *The Condition of Postmodernity*, Oxford: Blackwell.

Hekman, S.J. (1995) *Moral Voices, Moral Selves*, Cambridge: Polity Press.

Hodgkin, P. (1996) 'Medicine, postmodernism, and the end of certainty', *BMJ* 313: 1568–9.

Hume, D. (1975 [1777]) *Enquiries Concerning Human Understanding and Concerning the Principles of Morals*, Oxford: Oxford University Press.

Kuhn, T.S. (1970) *The Structure of Scientific Revolutions*, Chicago: University of Chicago Press.

Levinas, E. (1969) *Totality and Infinity*, Pittsburgh: Duquesne University Press.

Lyon, D. (1994) *Postmodernity*, Buckingham: Open University Press.

Lyotard, J.-F. (1984) *The Postmodern Condition: A Report on Knowledge*, Manchester: Manchester University Press.

Mathers, N. and Rowland, S. (1997) 'General practice – a postmodern speciality?', *British Journal of General Practice* 47: 177–9.

Norris, C. (1996) *Reclaiming Truth*, London: Lawrence and Wishart.

Porter, R. (1997) Introduction, in R. Porter (ed.) *Rewriting the Self*, London: Routledge.

Rorty, R. (1997) *Philosophy and the Mirror of Nature*, Princeton, NJ: Princeton University Press.

Silverman, H.J. (1993) Introduction in H.J. Silverman (ed.) *Questioning Foundations*, London: Routledge.

Smart, B. (1993) *Postmodernity*, London: Routledge.

Smith G.B. (1996) *Nietzsche, Heidegger and the Transition to Postmodernity*, Chicago: University of Chicago Press.

Tucket, D.A., Boulton, M., Olson, C. and Williams, A. (1985) *Meetings Between Experts: An Approach to Sharing Ideas in Medical Consultations*, London: Tavistock Publications.

Weinberg, S. (1993) *Dreams of Final Theory*, London: Vintage.

Part II

Topics

Chapter 7

The ethics of prescribing

Colin Bradley

INTRODUCTION – WHAT IS GOOD PRESCRIBING?

In 1990 the UK Department of Health launched the Indicative Prescribing Scheme. This was described in a document called 'Improving Prescribing' (Department of Health, 1990). Family Health Services Authorities, as they were then, were to appoint medical and pharmaceutical advisors charged with the task of improving general practitioners' prescribing. This description of their task presupposes that improvement is possible, which further implies that some prescribing was 'bad' and that other prescribing, by contrast, must be 'good'. What constitutes good prescribing was not defined, but it was taken to be synonymous with the concept of 'rational prescribing', an already well-established concept widely used as a basis for judging the quality of prescribing (Bradley, 1991). The use of the term 'rational prescribing' as a synonym for good prescribing also implies that good prescribing is a purely technical matter which involves comparing one's prescribing, or proposed prescribing, to a set of criteria. A relatively simple set of criteria proposed by Parish (1973) is widely accepted. He defined rational prescribing as prescribing that is appropriate, effective, safe and economic. Barber (1995) has highlighted the limitations of this over-simplified technical view. The terms 'safe' and 'effective' he suggests are absolutes that are rarely achievable. Our understanding of what is 'economic' has become more sophisticated with the development of the discipline of health economics. The meaning of 'appropriate' was always ambiguous and recent restatements of the definition of 'rational prescribing' either elaborate the term or omit it altogether. Furthermore, listing the criteria of rational prescribing fails to capture the reality of achieving 'good' patient care, which involves a complex balancing of these considerations. Barber suggests that, rather than judging prescribing per se, we ought to investigate what the prescriber was trying to achieve. He suggests the prescriber has four aims, namely:

- to maximize effectiveness;
- to minimize risk;
- to minimize cost;
- and to respect the patient's choices.

These aims can be seen as merely a restatement of the four ethical duties of all doctors espoused by deontological medical ethics (Beauchamp and Childress, 1994; Gillon, 1985) (see Table 1).

Table 1 **The correspondence between the Parish criteria for rational prescribing, Barber's aims of good prescribing and the principles of deontological medical ethics.**

Parish criterion for rational prescribing	Barber's aims for good prescribing	Deontological principle
Effective	To maximize effectiveness	Beneficence
Safe	To minimize risk	Non-maleficence
Economic	To minimize cost	Justice
Appropriate	To respect the patient's choice	Respect for autonomy

Also, as is recognized in the deontological approach to ethics, the challenge is not just in applying the underlying principles (viz. beneficence, non-maleficence, justice and respect for autonomy), but in balancing the principles where they conflict with one another. This account also highlights the fact that prescribing decisions are not purely technical ones, but always have an ethical dimension. The use of the word 'good' to describe prescribing carries with it an appropriate moral overtone that goes beyond the merely technical. This chapter will illustrate how medical ethics impinge, or ought to impinge, on prescribing in general practice and how the technical considerations involved in prescribing 'rationally' are inextricably bound up with the ethical issues of prescribing 'properly'.

NON-MALEFICENCE

The principle of non-maleficence is often summarized by the dictum '*primum non nocere*' (first do no harm). Adherence to this principle, in any absolute sense, though, is impossible because all medicines carry a potential for harming as well as healing the patient. Adverse effects span a very wide range from minor discomforts, such as the dry mouth commonly seen with many drugs, to life-threatening conditions such as aplastic anaemia. They include effects that can be predicted from the known pharmacological properties of the drug, but also effects that are only discovered with empirical experience in the use of the drug in patients and might include effects that are not yet known or reported. Finally, drugs may also affect people adversely because of interaction with other drugs that the patient is taking simultaneously. This is usually considered separately from other adverse effects in the technical medical literature but, from an ethical viewpoint, it is similar in that doctors are under the same moral obligation to avoid both interaction and adverse effects.

Ethically, therefore, doctors should be familiar with common adverse effects of drugs they prescribe and their common clinically significant interactions. They should also be aware of contra-indications to the use of drugs they prescribe and be alert to the presence of such contra-indications in patients they see. They are under greater moral obligation to ensure they avoid predictable adverse effects than they are to avoid effects that are unknown or unpredictable. The strength of this obligation is modulated by the seriousness of the possible adverse effect. In the case of drug interactions, a useful distinction might be drawn between interactions arising between two or more drugs the doctor has prescribed himself or herself and interactions between prescribed drugs and drugs obtained without the knowledge of the doctor such as 'street' drugs, social drugs (i.e. alcohol, caffeine, etc.) or over-the-counter medicines. Even in relation to such potentially 'unknown' drugs taken simultaneously, the degree of obligation on the doctor varies. Doctors might reasonably be expected to enquire about use of drugs purchased over the counter for the condition with which the patient has presented and possibly also for drugs taken contemporaneously for other reasons (Bradley and Bond, 1995). The obligation to try and avoid interaction with 'recreational' drugs may be considered to vary with the age of the patient (it would be more reasonably expected to make enquiries from younger patients who are known to be more likely to indulge in this behaviour) and with the practice setting (as in certain practice settings drug misuse is known to be common).

The duty to prescribe safely applies to all doctors but general practitioners have a requirement to be particularly safety conscious because general practice is a low risk environment from the point of view of morbidity. For a patient with any given symptom, such as headache, the probability of this being due to a serious disease are low. Similarly, the probability of the illness being due to a benign self-limiting disease is proportionately greater. This means that the use of a drug with a given (relatively constant) probability of causing a given adverse effect will, in a general practice setting, be more at risk of having undesired rather than the desired effects. The implications of this are that general practitioners ought to be more conservative than hospital colleagues in their prescribing of all drugs.

Technical aspects of drug safety

Ensuring drugs are safe is, of course, not the sole responsibility of the prescribing doctor. He or she is provided with guidance both from the manufacturers of the drugs and from a number of other independent sources. This guidance is based on the collected experience of use of the drug acquired initially through clinical trials and later through drug safety monitoring schemes such as the 'yellow card' scheme (Bateman and Chaplin, 1991). Manufacturers are obliged, under the terms of their licence to market the product, to provide any safety information of which they are aware concerning a drug they are selling. The format this guidance must take is regulated. This is now called the Summary of Product Characteristics (SPC). It was previously known as the Data Sheet (Association of the British Pharmaceutical Society, 1996). The SPCs of all prescription drugs are sent to doctors annually. The SPC should accompany any promotional material given or sent to doctors including adverts (in which an abbreviated version is allowed). Of course, with such guidance so readily available, prescribers are under a moral, and indeed legal, responsibility to follow the guidance unless a strong case can be made for not following it. Reliance on one's own experience of a drug, particularly for general practitioners, would not usually be adequate evidence to justify ignoring the official guidance.

All the adverse reactions associated with a drug are not necessarily known at the time of licensing. The duty of care of all doctors to the population at large, i.e. the principle of justice, obliges doctors to report any adverse effects or interactions not previously known. The magnitude of the risk of adverse effects of a drug is better determined when reporting is more complete. Risks are more difficult to quantify accurately for newer drugs of which there is, necessarily, less experience and, hence, the duty on doctors to report adverse effects is that much greater again. In the UK, in various sources of drug information (e.g. the British National Formulary, the Drug and Therapeutics Bulletin and MIMS), newer drugs are designated with an inverted black triangle (▼). For drugs carrying this symbol the Committee on the Safety of Medicines asks that doctors report any adverse reactions whether previously reported or not. This request carries with it a degree of moral obligation based on the ethical principles of non-maleficence and justice, i.e. ensuring the safety of both current and future patients.

Use of unlicensed drugs and drugs beyond the terms of their licence

General practitioners may occasionally be asked to prescribe an unlicensed drug. More commonly, in clinical practice medicines are used for purposes beyond those specified in the product licence. Manufacturer's guidance, if any, will usually be in the form of a disclaimer which warns the prescriber to weigh risks with benefits and treatment and make his or her own decision. This is just a restatement of the standard duty of the doctor in all prescribing. Before using a drug for an unlicensed indication or to use an unlicensed product, the doctor would be advised to seek guidance. Published, ideally peer reviewed, evidence and expert colleagues would be appropriate sources of advice. Ferner (1996) describes the obligations on the doctor in these circumstances. He discusses the different factors that might influence a decision to prescribe and offers a hierarchy of 'reasonableness of a prescribing decision'. This covers: patient factors (such as the age and gravid state or otherwise of the patient); illness factors (related to how serious the illness is from which the patient is suffering); drug factors (related to what is already known about the drug's safety profile); and factors relating to the reliability of sources of information about the proposed use of the drug and the licensed status of the drug. He also offers the sensible advice that any decision to use a drug beyond or outside its licence and the rationale for doing so should be carefully documented (see figure 1).

The legal position

The duty of non-malevolence on doctors has legal backing enshrined in the law of tort. This specifies the obligations on providers of services towards recipients of those services and provides for remedies where there is negligence. For negligence to be proven at law there are three requirements. It must be established that:

- the defendant had a duty of care towards the plaintiff;
- there was neglect of that duty;
- and that damage to the plaintiff resulted from that neglect.

Figure 1 Factors influencing the perceived reasonableness of prescribing decisions

	THE PATIENT	THE ILLNESS	THE DRUG	PUBLISHED DATA	STATUS*
Most reasonable					
↓	Young adult	Life-threatening	Well-known; generally safe	Recommended in standard textbooks	A
	Elderly		Well-known but some clear adverse effects	Well-documented studies in peer-reviewed journals	
	Child	Severe			B
	Breast-feeding†		Well-known; has serious adverse effects *or* Little-studied; no clear adverse effects	Only poor-quality studies reported	
	Infant	Mild			C
	Premenopausal woman		Little-studied; has serious adverse effects	Only anecdotal evidence published	
	Late pregnancy				
↓	Early pregnancy	Trivial	Not studied	No published data available	D
Least reasonable					

Source: From *Prescribers' Journal*, 36(2), 1996. Crown copyright is reproduced with the permission of the Controller of Her Majesty's Stationery Office.

Notes:

* Status A: Licensed for the intended indication.

* Status B: Licensed for another indication; other related products licensed for the intended indication.

* Status C: A licensed product; not licensed for the intended indication, nor are similar medicines.

* Status D: Drug/product not licensed at all.

† Mother, not infant.

In legal parlance, what is required is the exercise of 'due care', though what constitutes 'due care' is often difficult to define and is constantly being refined by case law. Under a common law system, such as prevails in Britain, the standard for 'due care' is derived from a consensus of what one's professional peers would regard as reasonable – a principle known as the 'Bolam principle'. Of course, such a consensus rarely exists *a priori* and often it has to be established on a case by case basis from opinions offered by expert witnesses called by each side in legal cases. Until recently, it was difficult for general practitioners to be construed, simultaneously, as professional peers and expert witnesses. However, the development of general practice as an academic discipline has enabled some general practitioners to be viewed by the courts as capable of being regarded as expert peers. This means that standards of 'due care' for general practice are effectively being defined by academics, as has, traditionally, been the case for other medical disciplines. Developments in academic general practice and, in particular, the guidelines for practice emanating from academic general practice research increasingly have legal and, arguably, ethical force.

Unintended effects and the rule of double effect

It has been noted above that drugs can sometimes cause adverse effects or have interactions that were previously unknown or could not have been predicted. If such adverse effects or interactions occur the doctor cannot reasonably be held legally or morally responsible. However, it is more often the case that doctors are obliged to prescribe drugs in spite of the known risks in order to derive the desired benefits. In this case the good effect of the drug can only be obtained if some exemption is granted from the '*primum non nocere*' maxim. A means of overcoming this difficulty, developed by Roman Catholic moral theologians, is known as the 'rule of double effect'. In its fullest statement it stipulates four conditions to be met for an act with double effect (i.e. both good and bad consequences) to be permitted:

- the action is good in itself (or at least morally neutral);
- the intention is solely to produce the good effect;
- the good effect is not achieved through the bad effect;
- and there is sufficient reason to permit the bad effect, i.e. that the good effect must outweigh the bad effect.

Many ethicists are highly critical of the rule of double effect and only die hard absolutists or theologians would insist on all the conditions being fulfilled in all instances. A quintessential double effect situation arises in terminal care when a decision has to be made about giving morphine to a patient to relieve pain (the good consequence) when the morphine might hasten death (the bad consequence). In this case, fulfilling the rule of double effect is usually possible and morphine may be given. However, there are many more instances in medical practice where clearly bad actions have to be taken, or the intention is to produce the bad effect as well as the good, or the good effect is not achievable except through the bad. For instance, the use of chemotherapy in cancer treatment might be difficult to justify under all the conditions of the rule of double effect. Even in the morphine example, many doctors might find they are rather more equivocal about their 'intentions' than is allowed for in the rule of double effect. The whole question of intent is a rather thorny one in medical ethics. The concept of intent has an honourable history in the development of moral philosophy and has recognition in legal process. Intent, though, can never be proven and accepting the role of intent runs the risk of providing a loophole for moral laxity or ineptitude. For double effect actions where the double effect is appreciated in advance it is difficult to sustain an argument of non-intentionality of the bad effect. A division of effects into desired and undesired might be more appropriate, though this is just a semantic resolution of the problem of intent. The rule of double effect is useful, though, in making us question all aspects of double effect actions, which virtually amounts to all prescribing. As a minimum, we should ensure that any adverse effects of an action are at least outweighed by the beneficial effects. It certainly rules out the exploitation of the adverse effects of drugs for other ends such as the case of the doctor who justified prescribing antibiotics for upper respiratory tract infection in the hope that the patient would get diarrhoea and learn not to ask for them again.

BENEFICENCE

Beneficence is sometimes seen as merely the opposite of non-maleficence – doing good as opposed to doing harm. However, the term beneficence has implications that go beyond the simple avoidance of harm to others, a virtually universal requirement of ethical behaviour in all spheres of life. The principle of beneficence encompasses preventing harm, removing harm and actively promoting good. With regard to prescribing, the minimum requirement of beneficence is that the doctor should prescribe drugs that are efficacious for the condition being treated – tempered, of course, by the need to avoid harm. It precludes the use of drugs that are known, or believed, by the doctor to have no specific therapeutic benefit. Some doctors would argue that there are no such drugs, as even pharmacologically inert substances have been shown to have beneficial effects (in about a third of instances in most studies) mediated by the placebo effect (Brody, 1977). The use of placebos in a therapeutic context, though, is morally suspect because they may be an affront to a person's autonomy (see below). The use of a drug with an effect demonstrably better than a placebo may still be a breach of the principle of beneficence if there are drugs for the same condition which have a demonstrably greater efficacy. Applying the beneficence principle is not simply about doing good but is, rather, about doing the maximum good possible. Thus the principle of beneficence requires that one should use the most effective drug for the condition being treated, although this may have to be tempered by the principle of justice if the more effective drug is more expensive (see below). Similarly, we are required not just to do good but to do that which would create the most good. The concept of maximizing good is a principal tenet of utilitarianism. Utilitarianism, indeed, can be construed so as to subsume the deontological principles being espoused here (Gillon, 1985).

Efficacy and evidence-based medicine

The minimum requirement is that doctors should only prescribe drugs that are efficacious. What constitutes efficacy, though, is not a simple matter of whether or not the drug 'works' in a pharmacological sense, although this is an important starting point. The determination of whether or not a drug 'works' usually takes place in a clinical trial. Drugs that do not satisfy the licensing authority that they 'work' in this sense will not be licensed. We often encounter patients, however, who do not exactly match those included in the trial and who nonetheless need to be treated. This requires doctors to judge whether or not the patient is a sufficiently close match to those in the trial for the trial result to be reasonably likely to be replicated in this patient. (See Chapter 2 on evidence-based medicine.) Various factors in the patient may decrease this probability. These factors do have to be judged carefully for, if the probability of accruing a similar benefit to that described in the trial is too low, it may be wrong (i.e. unethical) to prescribe the drug. Patients with milder disease than those included in the trial, patients with co-existing disease (especially disease likely to affect drug metabolism and make the risk of drug toxicity greater), patients who are older or younger than those in the trial, and patients who could be pregnant are at reduced probability of accruing a net benefit from use of the drug.

Other features of the trial may also be important in determining how much prescribers can rely on the results. Sometimes a single trial will not have amassed enough information of sufficient reliability to answer clinical questions about the use of a given drug. Results from several trials may have to be combined in order to decide what to do. A rigorous technique for doing this, known as meta-analysis, has been evolved. Judging the quality of clinical trials and meta-analyses are part of the emerging concept of evidence-based medicine (Sackett *et al.*, 1997).

Evidence-based medicine has its critics, who protest that there is more to clinical decision making than compiling and applying research evidence (Sweeney, 1996). However, to avoid discovering or to refuse to be guided by the best scientific evidence available is arguably unethical. To maximize good one must at least find and make use of the best evidence available.

Prescribing under uncertainty

While some poor prescribing may be done in ignorance of or in defiance of the best evidence available, it is, perhaps, more often the case that the best evidence is not adequate to the clinical decision which must be taken. There may not be a good quality trial and one may have to be guided by poor quality trials. The patient may not fit the categories used in the trial(s), but may still be sufficiently similar in terms of the condition being suffered to mean the treatment should be actively considered at least. Or it may be that there are no trials of the treatment for the condition, in which case an effort must be made to weigh risks and benefits using the best information available. Formal techniques to reduce this type of uncertainty, such as probability theory and decision analysis, are described in Chapter 1. These, though, are impractical in short GP consultations and some medical ethicists reject decision analysis as too mechanistic and insensitive to the patient's perspective (Pellegrino and Thomasma, 1988). However, the philosophy underlying decision analysis and principle elements of the approach do have something to offer when trying to make difficult decisions in the absence of complete information or when seeking to individualize treatment on the basis of information derived from populations. Thus, in prescribing decisions, one should ensure that all viable options are considered and that one's perceptions of the probabilities of harm and benefit accord with whatever up-to-date clinical trial evidence is available. While formal measurement of patient's utilities, i.e. the value they place on the various possible outcomes, will not usually be feasible, an effort should be made to ascertain the patient's view of the risks and benefits. Great care is required in how information on the probabilities of risks and benefits and the margins of error of our knowledge of these is presented to patients (Tversky and Kahneman, 1981). On the one hand, patients must be given full and unbiased information sufficient to make their choice within the limitations of their willingness and ability to receive and comprehend such information (see below, pp. 120–1). On the other hand, doctors must not abrogate their responsibilities to either assist patients make choices or make choices for patients when it is appropriate to do so.

Effectiveness and health gain

The ultimate aim of all therapy, of course, is not so much that the drug will 'work' in a purely pharmacological sense, but that overall the patient's condition improves or, to put it in the modern parlance, that there is a net 'health gain' for the patient. The measurement of health gain is even more difficult than the measurement of pharmacological efficacy (Metcalfe, 1990). It requires an ability to measure the health status of the patient, i.e. how healthy the person is in some overall sense, and to compare health status over time. Following a course of treatment or a health intervention there should be a change in health status, ideally towards a more favourable one. Clearly, side effects or undesirable effects of intervention reduce the net health gain from the intervention, even one that 'works', i.e. is efficacious. However, other factors affect health gain, or apparent health gain, too. Health status, even in the absence of interventions, fluctuates over time, with an overall tendency to decline with age. Many diseases wax and wane. Many measures of health gain are either so broad that they are insensitive to small changes in function or capacity brought about by health care interventions, or they are so specific that they cannot be used to compare different treatments which act on different aspects of the global experience of ill health. What is possibly more important than the technical measurement of health gain, from the point of view of a general practitioner, is the concept of looking for overall improvement in the patient's condition rather than whether or not the drug prescribed has had the predicted effect.

Beneficence and paternalism

Beneficence, particularly when formulated to incorporate non-maleficence, is held by some to be the overriding principle in medical ethics (Pellegrino and Thomasma, 1988). Beneficence can also be discerned as the main principle in most oaths, declarations and codes that have been used over the centuries to guide or stipulate the expected behaviour of doctors (Gillon, 1985). However, objections to this formulation of medical ethics have been based on the charge that giving such overriding priority to beneficence leads to paternalism. The acceptability or otherwise of paternalism in medicine relates to the issue of autonomy (see below). While, historically, medical practice was based on an assumption of diminished autonomy of patients (in so far as the patient's autonomy was considered relevant at all), this is no longer an acceptable assumption. Indeed, it has never been a safe assumption for the majority of patients and is particularly not so for most patients seen in general practice. In general practice the patient can nearly always assert their autonomy by not adhering to the management proposed by the doctor. Given that patients will do what they want whatever a doctor wishes, it is better not to adopt a paternalistic stance when prescribing treatment. We should aim to achieve 'concordance' between doctor and patient in prescribing and medicines use (Royal Pharmaceutical Society of Great Britain, 1997). The term 'concordance' was coined by a working party of the Royal Pharmaceutical Society of Great Britain that examined the problem of non-compliance with or non-adherence to prescribed regimens of treatment (McGavock, 1996). Embedded in this new term is the concept that what is required for successful medicine taking is a negotiation between equals and the formation of a therapeutic alliance between them. This clearly rules out paternalism as a route to beneficence.

RESPECT FOR AUTONOMY

Autonomy is a complex concept deriving from the Greek autos (self) and nomos (rule) which, in reference to individuals, has two essentials elements. First, the idea of liberty, i.e. independence from external control or influence, and second, the notion of a capacity for independent action. In the context of health care, in contrast to the legal situation, people are not either autonomous or non-autonomous but rather have a variable capacity to act autonomously depending on circumstances and the decision to be made or action to be taken. In medical care carefully considered judgements need to be made regarding whether or not, with respect to any particular intervention, the person for whom it is intended is capable of making an autonomous decision. The principle of respect for autonomy requires both an attitude of wishing to work with an autonomous person to assist them in making health care choices, but also requires actions to enhance that person's autonomy to whatever extent this is possible. As illness can, of itself, diminish people's autonomy the effective treatment of illness is a route to the enhancement of autonomy.

Informed consent

One of the important corollaries of respect for autonomy is the requirement to seek the informed consent of patients to treatment. This is, of course, also a legal requirement. Most of the time in primary care consent is implied rather than explicit. This presupposes that the patient's implied consent is informed. Consent to history taking and examination may well be informed by the patient's previous experience of the sort of things doctors do and why they do them. When it comes to taking medicine patients are much more at risk of lacking the necessary information to give (implied) informed consent. When prescribing, therefore, information may have to be provided first and consent to the treatment sought explicitly.

In practical terms, obtaining fully informed consent in all instances is virtually impossible, especially in the generally short consultation times typical of general practice. One way around this is to argue for a 'relational ethic' in which the ground rules for the relationship establish the patient's autonomy automatically (Brody, 1987). Thus, rather than having to seek explicit consent or inform the patient comprehensively, the relationship is conducted in such a way that it is clear to the patient that he or she is free to interrupt at any time and seek any information he or she requires. The doctor, it is then supposed, can proceed efficiently with treatment without the need to check each and every point of detail with the patient. This relational ethic is particularly appropriate to the longitudinal relationships typically seen in general practice. The idea that ethical rules for the doctor's conduct should be built into the relationship with the patient can be accepted readily. This does not, however, displace the need for a decisional ethic to prevail as well and for each decision to be capable of being judged on its merits, admittedly informed by what has preceded it in the relationship.

This still leaves the question of what would constitute adequately informed consent to treatment in the ordinary general practice consultation. (See Chapter 3 for a detailed consideration of consent.) As a minimum, patients ought to be told the name of the drug or drugs the doctor is proposing to prescribe; what the drug (s) are supposed to do for the patient; how and when they are to be taken; and for how long they are to be taken. In addition, common adverse effects ought, in most instances, to be notified to the patient and the extent to which the doctor sees the medicines as essential to health or merely symptom relieving should also be clarified (see Box 1).

Box 1 A suggested minimum information set for informed consent to prescribing in general practice

- The name of the drug or drugs
- What the drug (s) are supposed to do
- How and when they are to be taken
- How long they are to be taken for
- Common adverse effects and interactions
- Extent to which the medicines are (believed by the doctor to be) essential to health

Information to be provided above and beyond this ought to be at the patient's discretion rather than the doctor's and information, including that about side effects, should not be unreasonably withheld. Furthermore, patients must be given an opportunity within the consultation to ask their questions about the proposed treatment (s) and it should be made clear to them that they are free to make contact at any later time should they have any questions about their treatment (s). Where there is a degree of uncertainty about the treatment – either its efficacy, safety or appropriateness – respect for autonomy would demand that this uncertainty is also shared with the patient. Sharing of uncertainty, though, may have to be tempered by considerations of beneficence as in therapeutic privilege (see below). The nature of the uncertainty (see Chapter 1) ought to be shared also. This will clearly be uncomfortable for doctors, particularly where the source of their uncertainty is their own ignorance. However, patients are more tolerant of ignorance on the part of their doctors than doctors tend to give them credit for. They might become more tolerant still if such declarations of personal ignorance were more the norm (as they should be – no doctor can know everything even about his/her own field). Besides, morally speaking, ignorance is less culpable than dishonesty. More discomfort about our personal ignorance might also spur us to lessen that ignorance, which would itself be a good thing for our patients.

Intentional non-disclosure

The above implies that informed consent is a *sine qua non* of medical treatment and that full disclosure (or at least as full as is necessary for the patient and as is feasible) is a necessary corollary of respect for autonomy. There are, however, circumstances under which non-disclosure is held to be permissible. The first of these relates to the concept of 'therapeutic privilege' which actually enjoys some recognition within the legal requirements of informed consent. Where a doctor judges that disclosure might harm the patient it may be permissible for the doctor to proceed with treatment without the need to fully inform the patient of all its consequences (or potential consequences). For instance, if telling a patient about all the risks of a potentially life-saving drug might lead to his refusing it one might, at least temporarily, hold back some of the information under therapeutic privilege. The notion of therapeutic privilege is under attack in modern ethical thinking and now it is a privilege which needs to be deployed, if at all, under much more stringent conditions. The gains from non-disclosure must be very clear and the losses (including to patient autonomy) must be minimized.

The second instance relates to the case of the therapeutic use of placebos. First, it has been claimed that it is possible to achieve the placebo effect without the need for a placebo per se. In one study it was found that patients still benefited from a placebo pill even though they had been told openly that it was a placebo (Park *et al.*, 1967). Its use was justified to the patients on the basis that other patients with symptoms similar to theirs had benefited in about 30 per cent of instances. Others argue that the placebo effect is not one of the actual placebo substance but is rather a product of the 'healing context' and thus is possible to achieve without the need for either deception or, indeed, anything that resembles a medicine (Brody, 1977; Balint, 1964). However, placebos are less likely to work with the patient's knowledge and so it is possible to visualize extreme cases in which their use might be justified. Such non-disclosure is still an affront to the patient's autonomy and so must be strongly justified on other grounds such as beneficence.

Pure and impure placebos

Pharmacologically inert substances deployed for their psychological effects, as in clinical trials, are 'pure placebos'. 'Impure' or 'pseudo placebo' use occurs where a drug with known active pharmacological properties is deployed more for its placebo effects (which all drugs have) than for its proper pharmacological action. This use of drugs, though widespread, is morally reprehensible. A common instance in general practice is the use of antibiotics for upper respiratory tract infections (see below) in which the antibiotic is given because the patient is said to expect it and it will, presumably, have a placebo effect. Not only does this deny the patient's autonomous right to be informed of the nature and purpose of treatment but it risks breaching the principle of non-maleficence as well. Harm may occur through side effects of the active pharmacological substance or by medicalizing the problem (Little *et al.*, 1997).

Paradoxically, meeting patients' expectations is often justified as respecting their autonomy. Patients expectations, though, are a mixture of what the patient anticipates will happen and what he/she hopes will happen (Britten, 1995). A simplistic view of patients' aspirations would hold that, particularly when these are vocalized within the consultation, they are an expression of a patient's autonomy and ought to be met in all but exceptional circumstances. However, if patients' expectations are properly probed one usually finds patients do not want the medicine *per se* but they want the benefits they believe the medicine will bring. The patient may, of course, be right and the medicine might be reasonably expected to provide the benefit legitimately sought. In this case, the patient's wishes should certainly be granted. Patient's wishes are more often ill informed or based on short-term rather than long-term ideas of benefit. Occasionally, a patient's aspirations are not based on medical needs at all but are socially driven, as in wanting to have the same treatment as a friend or social rival. In these cases the doctor is not obliged to concede to requests. The proper way of dealing with a patient's requests where these do not accord with the doctor's view of what is best for the patient is beyond the scope of this book and has been dealt with by this author elsewhere (Bradley, 1994). It is worth noting that the underlying problem in these cases stems from the power imbalance in the doctor–patient relationship. The power imbalance is intrinsic to the relationship and yet it diminishes the patient's relative autonomy. The principle of respect for autonomy requires that doctors work to reduce the power imbalance in their relationships with patients and, similarly, that they should not exploit the power imbalance deliberately even when this might appear justified on beneficent grounds.

JUSTICE

Of all the ethical concepts relevant to medical practice the concept of justice is, perhaps, the most complex. At its heart, however, is the straightforward and intuitively understood concept of fairness usually expressed as 'equals must be treated equally and unequals unequally'. Material or substantive principles of justice establish the basis on which equality or inequality is to be judged. The principles of justice developed in the health care system focus almost exclusively on distributive justice, i.e. the sharing out of health care resources. When it comes to allocating health care resources the question of which material principles of justice are valid, i.e. which inequalities are relevant, is highly contentious. Allocating health care on a same share to each person basis seems intuitively illogical when applied to individuals although modifications of the principle have been proposed for distribution of resources at higher (e.g. regional) levels (Draper and Tunna, 1996). An allocation on the basis of medical need is probably the most traditional principle and the one preferred by many doctors. However, what constitutes medical need is not a simple matter and this alone fails to consider the effectiveness treatment. If the potential for medical success is taken into consideration one comes closer to a utilitarian or welfare maximization view. This, in turn, ignores the 'rule of rescue' which Hadorn (1992) defines as 'the strong human proclivity to provide aid to identified victims of illness and accident'. Overt utilitarianism also leads to explicit rationing which is deeply unpopular. Furthermore, even when need is clearly defined, there may still not be sufficient resources to meet all the need identified and other principles may come into play, such as merit or social worth. Merit, for instance, can be accorded to patients depending on whether or not they are seen as having contributed to their own ill health. This sort of consideration has been invoked more often as a basis for denying treatment than for providing it as in the controversy over whether or not to provide coronary artery bypass surgery to patients who smoke.

Economics and prescribing

When it comes to prescribing, the main way in which justice considerations intrude is through the need to prescribe economically. This is because of the economic concept of opportunity costs which dictates that resources expended in one area of, say, health care are unavailable for expenditure elsewhere – this is simply a corollary of the indisputable fact that, ultimately, resources are always limited. The implication for prescribing is that if one prescribes a more expensive drug less money is available for expenditure on other goods. For GPs who participate in fundholding or commissioning schemes, the link between treatments provided to one patient leading to other treatments being denied other patients is made starkly obvious. Justice demands that the treatment used should be the least expensive that will achieve the required benefit for the patient. Furthermore, relatively expensive treatments (such as IVF, see below) that may be justifiable on an individual basis become harder to justify on a population basis. Even for lower cost treatments additional facets of the treatment that do not add to its efficacy, such as greater palatability, should not come into consideration. However, these seemingly minor aspects of treatment may, for an individual patient, be a major determinant of whether or not he or she takes the medicine at all. Needless to say, a medicine not taken properly is an even greater waste of resources. What is required to square this circle is a greater effort to achieve concordance with the patient (see above) and a restriction of more expensive medicines to cases where their greater expense is justified.

Another economic concept of some importance is that of diminishing returns. This principle indicates that for each additional patient treated along a continuum of patients from the most ill to the least ill the health gain is less and, hence, harder to justify economically and, hence, ethically. The reason this usually applies to medical treatments is that the marginal benefit of each additional patient treated may not be balanced by the marginal cost (i.e. the cost of each additional patient treated). While this may not hold for treatments requiring a substantial capital outlay, it is certainly true of prescribing where the bulk of any marginal cost is made up by the cost of the drugs which, of course, are usually fixed. This has particular relevance for primary care physicians because proportionately more of our patients are less ill. Hence, a treatment that may make economic sense for a hospital patient may not be economically justified when applied to the majority of community-based ambulatory patients. This argument applies particularly well to drug costs but, of course, drugs are only part of treatment and costs are not always purely financial. Another important resource in general practice is the doctor's time and, with this resource, one has to be careful that the diminishing returns argument is not too readily invoked. Sometimes a little extra time spent with a patient, particularly early on in the doctor–patient relationship, can repay considerable benefits to that patient, sufficient to justify the cost of waiting for other patients. When this applies, though, it is a matter requiring considerable clinical judgement.

TWO ILLUSTRATIVE CASES

So far in this chapter what has been presented are the ethical arguments which support the criteria for 'good' prescribing. The chapter has emphasized that many of the technical considerations in prescribing have an ethical dimension and, hence, are backed, to an extent, by a moral imperative. However, the very essence of ethics, particularly as seen from a deontological stance, is that ethical difficulties and decisions arise precisely because all the relevant moral imperatives cannot be satisfied. Inevitably, one has to choose among the apparent imperatives to which to give priority. Balancing considerations of beneficence and non-malevolence is fairly familiar to doctors. Less familiar, though rising up the ethical agenda, are conflicts between beneficence/non-malevolence and respect for autonomy and conflicts between beneficence/non-malevolence and justice. Two cases are presented which highlight these conflicts and indicate an approach to their resolution.

The case of antibiotics for upper respiratory tract infection – A conflict between beneficence/non-malevolence and respect for autonomy

A mother brings her 12-year-old daughter to the surgery with a four-day history of upper respiratory tract symptoms of cough productive of whitish sputum, sore throat, fever and coryza. She has no wheeze or history of recurrent respiratory problems. History and physical examination confirm a diagnosis of simple upper respiratory tract infection. The mother says that she brought her daughter along so you 'could give her a course of antibiotics'. Should you prescribe the antibiotics requested?

Beneficence/non-maleficence

The antibiotics will almost certainly make the mother feel better. She will be reassured both that her request was taken seriously and that active treatment of the problem has been undertaken. Everything that can be done is being done, she supposes. The antibiotics are likely to have a placebo effect, which may be quite strong as antibiotics are perceived as very powerful medicines. The antibiotics may even treat a covert or incipient bacterial infection if one happens to co-exist. If care is taken to exclude allergies to the antibiotics, serious side effects are rare. Other commoner side effects, such as diarrhoea or rashes, may occur but many doctors dismiss these side effects as inconsequential. Some doctors may even hope their occurrence might encourage patients to desist from requesting antibiotics for minor infections.

Respect for autonomy

Acceding to the direct patient request for a treatment that is seen as not unreasonable and is fairly innocuous, it is argued, shows respect for the freely expressed and autonomous wish of the patient. Contrariwise, to deny the treatment may be seen as unjustified paternalism. However, to pretend that the antibiotics are working via a specific pharmacological effect when, in fact, the doctor is relying primarily on their pseudo placebo effect involves deceit of the patient, which is an affront to her autonomy. This case is additionally complicated by the age of the child, which is such that she cannot be assumed to be completely incapable of expressing a degree of autonomy. While a case could be made for ignoring the wishes of the child and relying on the mother to allow the child's autonomy to be expressed, an optimal position would seek to involve the child, within her capabilities, in any decision making.

Justice

Antibiotics prescribed unnecessarily are a waste of resources that could be reallocated to other patients in greater need. If the antibiotic prescribed is fairly cheap the cost of such prescribing may be seen as inconsequential in the greater scheme of things. The problem of antibiotic resistance means that prescribing them where not strictly indicated risks increasing the danger to other patients of antibiotic resistant strains of bacteria which, in ethical terms, is unjust. However, many general practitioners feel that this risk is exaggerated and that in a primary care setting the risk of antibiotic resistance is minimal. Furthermore, this scenario may be seen by many general practitioners as one in which expenditure of that other resource, viz. doctor's time, is not rewarded. Time spent trying to convince a reluctant patient, perhaps ultimately unsuccessfully, to go without antibiotics may be unjust from the point of view of other patients kept waiting.

Resolution

It should be clear from what has been said above regarding the need for general practitioners to be conservative in their use of drugs – general practice being a low risk environment, the undesirability of pseudo placebo use and so on – that prescribing antibiotics in this situation is ethically, as well as technically, undesirable. Consideration of each of the ethical issues may highlight the extent to which technical issues are, as yet, unresolved. For example, a review by the International Primary Care Network has highlighted how, in relation to otitis media at least, the technical issues are both complex and incompletely resolved (Froom *et al.*, 1997). However, the fact that such decisions are underpinned by ethical considerations makes it clear that there can be circumstances or facets to the case that, exceptionally, justify their use on non-technical grounds. For instance, if the mother of the child had had another child who had died of meningitis and had acquired a belief, maybe even a delusional belief, that antibiotics in this situation were the only available safeguard against meningitis, it would be cruel and unethical to deny her child antibiotics. Considering this case in an ethical framework highlights the importance of entering into a dialogue with the patient about their beliefs and aspirations so that a negotiation may take place that may still lead to her acceptance of the lack of utility of antibiotics.

The case of drugs for assisted fertility – a conflict between beneficence/non-malevolence and distributive justice

A couple, of modest means, in their mid-thirties, who have been trying to conceive for seven years, have been referred by you to the local infertility clinic. They have been told that the best chance of conception is by IVF (in vitro fertilization). This is not available on the NHS but is available from a private clinic. They have been to the clinic who sent them back to the practice to have the necessary drugs prescribed. They have had already three cycles of treatment prescribed by the practice at a cost of £2,000 per cycle. The practice, which is in the GP fundholding scheme, is already overspent. In discussion with the health authority, the practice agreed to curtail prescribing of drugs for assisted fertility, although the practice would not go along fully with the health authority's request to apply the authority's policy of obliging all patients to seek all such treatment from the private sector. The couple come requesting a prescription for another cycle of treatment. Should you prescribe the drugs requested?

Beneficence/non-maleficence

There are a number of significant technical issues in this case that have considerable impact on the ethical considerations. One of the major technical issues concerns the chances of success for any treatment undertaken. Another concerns the risks of treatment, particularly the risk of ovarian hyperstimulation. Leaving these aside and assuming the doctor is satisfied that, in purely technical terms, the risk–benefit relationship justifies treatment, there remain considerable ethical issues. There is still considerable debate possible around whether or not the automatic application of technological solutions to the problem of infertility is the correct approach. For instance, one major drawback to this approach is that it may delay or prevent the natural grieving process that would occur were the couple to decide to just accept their infertility, as had to be done before the availability of in vitro fertilization techniques. This argument against treatment is considerably strengthened if one takes the view that success rates of treatment are only very modest.

Respect for autonomy

A straightforward view of autonomy that only considers the expressed wishes of the couple might see no great problem with acceding to a request for treatment given that the doctor fulfils his or her duty under the terms of 'informed consent'. However, if one accords autonomy to embryos, as many theocentric views of ethical issues would, the issue arises as to whose autonomy is paramount. The fact that embryos may be produced that will not be 'used' immediately, if ever, further complicates the issues.

Justice and resolution

This sort of case, more clearly than many others, brings home to general practitioners their role as arbitrators of distributive justice. As fundholders, the GPs have a responsibility to see resources allocated fairly and yet as beneficent physicians they would want to see this couple achieve their eagerly sought goal. The £2,000 spent on this couple's next treatment cycle is £2,000 less for the practice fund for outpatient treatment which could, for instance, translate into six months of pain and additional suffering for a succession of arthritis sufferers awaiting hip replacement. This raises difficult questions as to which case deserves priority. The old gentleman with his arthritic hip has done his bit for society and now deserves the resources of society to be applied to his problem (a merit-based case). Yet this couple, if treatment is postponed, may become too old for successful treatment and so deserve priority (a welfare maximization argument). There is no easy way to resolve such issues. A better understanding of the technical issues and a recognition that there comes a point at which helping the couple to adapt to childlessness may be better, even for them, than repeatedly raising and dashing hopes may help us find a solution. In the end a common, and reasonable, solution is to set some limit on the number of treatment cycles to be allowed from public funds. Three would be regarded by many as a reasonable allocation. However, in this case, such a limit was not, perhaps, understood at the outset and to introduce it now may seem rather arbitrary and harsh. So, a case might be made for them of allowing one more cycle. This, of course, may run the risk of creating a precedent which would be difficult to resist in other cases were it to be successful and the fact that it was a fourth cycle to become well known in the practice population. It may also still not seem fair to the elderly arthritis sufferer. What is needed is a better system of public consultation about health resource allocation but, for now, doctors still have to take the difficult decisions. This does not preclude the possibility of involving current patients in those decisions. One can often be surprised by the willingness of some patients to forego expensive treatments when the opportunity cost concept is explained to them. Virtue is not confined to doctors and ethical duties, such as to justice, are not unique to us either.

CONCLUSIONS

This chapter began with a discussion of the concept of 'good' prescribing and illustrates how this is related to the technical issues of 'rational' prescribing. It has gone beyond these to incorporate moral values in the prescribing process. Although the technical issues underpin the actions that are required on ethical grounds, the two are not synonymous. This becomes particularly clear when one considers clinical cases where a technical or ethical case can be made for a decision to go either way, but the resolution of the difficulty requires ethical skills and not, necessarily, more technical knowledge.

KEY POINTS

- The technical requirements of rational prescribing are usually backed by an ethical imperative
- Non-maleficence requires safe prescribing
- Beneficence requires effective prescribing
- Respect for autonomy requires appropriate prescribing
- Justice requires economic prescribing
- Difficulties arise when two or more imperatives are in conflict
- Resolution usually requires ethical rather than technical judgements to be made

REFERENCES

Association of the British Pharmaceutical Industry (1996) *Compendium of Data Sheets and Summaries of Product Characteristics 1996–97*, London: Association of the British Pharmaceutical Industry.

Balint, M. (1964) *The Doctor, his Patient and the Illness*, 2nd edn, London: Pitman Medical.

Barber, N. (1995) 'What constitutes good prescribing?', *British Medical Journal* 310: 923–5.

Bateman, D.N. and Chaplin, S. (1991) 'Adverse reactions to drugs', in J. Feely (ed.) *New Drugs*, London: British Medical Journal.

Beauchamp, T.L. and Childress, J.F. (1994) *Principles of Biomedical Ethics*, 4th edn, Oxford: Oxford University Press.

Bradley, C.P. (1991) 'Decision making and prescribing patterns – a literature review', *Family Practice* 8: 276–85.

Bradley, C.P. (1994) 'Learning to say "No". An exercise in learning to decline inappropriate prescription requests', *Education for General Practice* 5: 112–19.

Bradley, C.P. and Bond, C. (1995) 'Increasing the number of drugs available over the counter: arguments for and against', *British Journal of General Practice* 45: 553–6.

Britten, N. (1995) 'Patients' demands for prescriptions in primary care'. *British Medical Journal* 310: 1084–5.

Brody, H. (1977) *Placebos and the Philosophy of Medicine: Clinical, Conceptual and Ethical Issues*, Chicago: University of Chicago Press.

Brody, H. (1987) *Stories of Sickness*, New Haven: Yale University Press.

Department of Health (1990) *Improving Prescribing*, London: HMSO.

Draper, H. and Tunna, K. (1996) *Ethics and Values for Commissioners*, Leeds: Nuffield Institute for Health.

Ferner, R. (1996) 'Prescribing licensed medicines for unlicensed indications'. *Prescribers' Journal* 36: 72–8.

Froom, J., Culpepper, L., Jacobs, M., DeMelker, R.A., Green, L.A., van Buchem, L., Grob, P. and Heeren, T. (1997) 'Antimicrobials for acute otitis media? A review from the International Primary Care Network', *British Medical Journal* 315: 98–102.

Gillon, R. (1985) *Philosophical Medical Ethics*, Chichester: John Wiley and Sons.

Hadorn, D.C. (1992)'The problem of discrimination in health care priority setting'. *Journal of the American Medical Association* 268: 1454–8.

Little, P., Gould, C., Williamson, I., Warner, G., Gantley, M. and Kinmonth, A.L. (1997) 'Reattendance and complications in a randomised trial of prescribing strategies for sore throat: the medicalising effect of prescribing antibiotics', *British Medical Journal* 315: 350–2.

McGavock, H. (1996) 'A review of the literature on drug adherence', London: Royal Pharmaceutical Society of Great Britain.

Metcalfe, D. (1990) 'Measurement of outcomes in general practice', in A. Hopkins and D. Costain (eds) *Measuring the Outcomes of Medical Care*, London: Royal College of Physicians.

Parish, P. (1973) 'Drug prescribing – the concern of all', *Journal of the Royal Society of Health* 93: 213–17.

Parkes, L.C. *et al.* (1967) 'Effects of informed consent on research patients and study results', *Journal of Nervous and Mental Disease* 145: 349–57.

Pellegrino, E.D. and Thomasma, D.C. (1988) 'Making decision under uncertainty', *For the Patient's Good. The Restoration of Beneficence in Health Care*, Oxford: Oxford University Press.

Royal Pharmaceutical Society of Great Britain (1997) *From Compliance to Concordance. Achieving Shared Goals in Medicine Taking*, London: Royal Pharmaceutical Society of Great Britain.

Sackett, D.L., Richardson, W.S., Rosenberg, W. and Haynes, R.B. (1997) *Evidence-Based Medicine. How to Practice and Teach EBM*, Edinburgh: Churchill Livingstone.

Sweeney, K. (1996) 'Evidence and uncertainty', in M. Marinkes (ed.) *Sense and Sensibility in Health Care*, London: British Medical Journal.

Tversky, A. and Kahneman, D. (1981) 'The framing of decisions and the psychology of choice', *Science* 211: 453–8.

Chapter 8

Depression in general practice

Roger Higgs

> 'Er, tha's got a reet black dog o' tha rigg this morning, lad. What's opp?'
>
> (West Riding Mill Foreman, 1959)

Churchill called it a black dog too. But though he and the darkly satanic Bradford woolmills have now gone, the black dog has not. Quite the reverse. From being something to hide or take to the confessional, depression is now often offered by patients as the open and opening reason for coming to see their GP. It is a subject of interest for the media and the general public, whether the glib chattering upper classes late at Saturday night dinner parties, or the teeth chattering working classes in early Monday morning bus queues. Why is this, and why should it be an issue for the general practitioner and her staff? The available answers, often pitting the escalating work load of a busy generalist against the distress of clients and the dangers they face, seem to make assumptions that fail to examine the moral dimension of this discussion.

To look at this discussion in any depth we shall have to ask further questions. What is depression and why is it so important? Are the moral questions it raises different from those raised overall within health care? How should we view it and how should we assess the responses general practice can offer? These and related questions may take us straight to the concepts commonly used in medical ethics discussions, such as respecting autonomy, avoiding harm or acting fairly, but may also take us beyond ethics to contested areas about the aims of medical care and the nature of mental illness. Some of these questions will be *ontological* questions – what sort of thing is the thing under discussion, what is its essence, in what way does it exist? – and touch on deeper *meta-ethical* problems, unanswerable here, about the nature of the good, meaning, difference and so on. If this appears to be unrelated to the clinical task, that of responding to the (perhaps umpteenth) distressed or miserable person in the consulting room, we shall test our ideas against the ways in which general practitioners see things, their particular values or mind set when they meet such people in a clinical encounter. And it will not be assumed that the only depressed person in such an encounter is the patient.

In Britain, general practice is one of the main parts of 'primary' health care, that is, the point where a person first declares himself or herself to be a patient and has, in a general sense in the NHS, open and free access to medicine. Thus, in spite of the attempt by practices to control and sort their workload by using appointment systems (in some ways a challenge to the 'open access' concept), the arithmetic of need and resource dictates that few GPs can offer more than a few minutes to each patient. Many patients coming to their GP are emotionally distressed in some way, whether largely so or in association with another illness or disease (Williams and Clare, 1979). Leaving aside the anxiety everyone must feel when going to the doctor, the exact nature of this distress may be hard for us to label, but many patients will be unhappy, tense or extremely sad. Some will be depressed in a way which any acute observer would recognize, and some (though by no means always the 'obviously' depressed) will be thinking of taking their lives. The risk of serious harm or loss of life brings the question of depression into sharp focus: not merely a question of suffering, but of survival. It is said that most who are suicidal visit their GP before the attempt – though the academic who played a late Beethoven quartet before going quietly to the carefully sealed garage, or the artist who posted her handbag at a seaside pillarbox before walking out through the waves to her death, raise the need for different kinds of awareness and approach. Some have questioned the mythology of the GP visit by every desperate person (Goldstein *et al.*, 1991). The equally mythical but general expectation of the GP as someone who will respond appropriately and promptly to any problem however presented creates anger in relatives and deep guilt in the practitioner when a patient dies by their own hand shortly after a consultation.

If the above is accepted as a realistic account, most readers will already have detected a clutch of practical and moral issues in the processes described which have to do with the service in general. Who controls the amount of professional time available and how is this costed? How could it be changed? The gatekeeper function of the GP already sets down an apparently paternalistic challenge to the concept of patient choice: what if as a patient I really want to see a specialist? There are more general questions which are beyond the scope of this chapter. But depression presents issues on its own account. Where is the borderline between distress and disease, between where medical services must intervene and where we wish they would if only they had the time or resources? Is moderate depression always an illness? If so, does it always need to be treated and in what way? Should the patient be able to choose how this is done or is it up to the professional? How will we judge on what basis this is assessed? More mundane problems may face a modernized practitioner with her computer screen facing the patient. The word itself, coldly typed on the screen, hardly seems to describe the desperation or despair some are telling; and what is written there may not help a person who later unthinkingly allows a life insurance company open access to these records. Yet this is perhaps to travel too far too fast. What can we be reasonably sure about in this area of mental health?

SOME CERTAINTIES OF DEPRESSION

The practice of ethics likes to ask questions, whereas the practice of medicine desperately needs answers. This can make the philosopher a valued companion, but not one always to take as a companion on a call at night or into a busy casualty, where decisions have to be made at speed, often on grossly inadequate evidence. But medicine need not be ashamed of its knowledge and clarities, painfully and painstakingly acquired through clinical practice and research, any more than is philosophy of the concepts and arguments which have equally as long and respected a lineage. Leaving aside the point of view of the complete sceptic, we can see a reasonable case being made for a number of certainties in a modern view of depression in both hospitals and general practice.

Depression is 'no respecter of persons' in the sixteenth-century sense: there is no class, occupation, ethnic group or personality type which is immune, and it may come to both sexes and all ages. On the other hand, there are some strong associations with adverse social and economic circumstances. The poor, the dispossessed, the unfortunate are at double peril; since their depression is all too understandable, they risk receiving no help for it, like the bereaved and terminally ill. It is somehow 'natural' and 'anyway, where would you stop?' There are probably useful distinctions to be made between a depression with whose cause we can empathise and one which comes like thunder out of a blue sky: this we shall need to return to. We may reflect on the statistics that 60–70 per cent of people who reach adult life will at some point experience depression or related symptoms severely enough to affect their ordinary lives and desired activities (Mann, 1992).

Although the diagnosis of depression as currently understood in medicine is not always easy, there is great unanimity as to what constitutes a 'case' and how this may be verified. Some of this may be as a result of subjective observation, but much depends on what the sufferer says, supplemented and validated as necessary by questionnaire instruments (see Box 1). Specialists in the field would claim that this makes a true diagnosis here as sure as any in medicine, even in the areas where a biopsy or a blood test can confirm a physical condition. More so, some might say, as the questionnaires make the judgement by reviewing the direct effect of such a state on the function of the patient, whereas the exceptional person with a high blood glucose or a liver half full of secondary cancer might still feel well enough to carry on life as normal until body systems became really dysfunctional. We can see here echoes of the inversion of conventional thinking achieved by Fulford in his ground-breaking work about mental and physical illness. His persuasive view is that since symptoms are perceived by and expressed in the mind, *illness* (subjective) emerges as the logically primary concept in medicine rather than *disease* (objective), and so by inference mental illnesses have as much if not more claim to be really the business of medicine as physical conditions (Fulford, 1989).

Box 1 Criteria for the diagnosis of major depression, as expressed in DSMIII-R

Five of the following must be present during the same fortnight period, and must include either depressed mood or diminished interest or pleasure.

1 Depressed mood
2 Greatly diminished interest in or pleasure from normal activities
3 Weight loss or gain (of significance)
4 Sleep disturbance
5 Feelings of excess guilt or worthlessness
6 Reduced ability to think or concentrate, or indecisiveness
7 Retardation or agitation
8 Fatigue or loss of energy
9 Recurrent thoughts of death or suicidal thoughts or actions

So depression is diagnosable: it is also important. Thousands of working days are lost because of people being depressed. If suicide is the outcome of the most serious forms (although we may need to re-examine the intrinsic circularities in this) and preventing preventable deaths one of doctors' clearest duties, then paying proper attention to depressed patients, or depression in people whom we come across, is well nigh an imperative.

But here we come face to face with a startling fact: doctors often miss it. Depression is now one of the common reasons for going to the doctor, and most people who get treated for it do so in the primary rather than secondary sector of health services (Freeling *et al.*, 1985). The figures on average indicate that up to half of the patients coming, for instance, to UK general practice may have symptoms of a low mood, and about one in twenty of these will have a major depression, as detailed in DSMIII-R criteria above (Freeling and Tylee, 1992; Bebbington *et al.*, 1981). This should make the primary care clinician an expert in picking up sufferers. Yet routinely it seems that only half are recognized by British GPs, even if some individuals report with much higher rates (Freeling *et al.*, 1985). So half the cases are going undetected, or at least unrecorded or unattended to, in many practices up and down the land. There is a rule of halves to be found elsewhere, for example in the detection and treatment of raised blood pressure (Wilber and Barrow, 1972), so perhaps this is not so shocking. However, hypertension is symptomless, by and large, whereas the depressed patient whose condition brings them to their doctor has real and, usually, vocalized complaints. There are claims that training can improve the detection rate, but this effect may not be lasting (Rutz *et al.*, 1992). What is clear is that there is a long way to go before a depressed Mrs Average has more than an evens chance of being diagnosed correctly or completely by busy Dr Mean.

From this point the sharp light of certainty begins to fade. It is possible that detecting and treating depression early may reduce the chances that it will persist (Scott *et al.*, 1992). The mixture of depressive with somatic symptoms reduces the likelihood of detection; many physically ill patients are depressed and vice versa. Other psychological states or conditions, like anxiety, substance abuse or dementia, likewise cloud the picture. There are claims that some of these will improve when proper or appropriate treatment for depression is given. But what is proper treatment? Thereby hangs a tale, 'and it may wag the dog'. Who decides on the best treatment and with what motives? What is clear, in sum, is that many ill people are depressed, and that many depressed people present as ill to their doctors; some make attempts on their lives. Those concerned feel a clear duty to make sure that the result is not silence.

THE CHALLENGE POSED BY ETHICS

There is hope that some of the uncertainties which remain can be dispelled by more, better or different research into the illness and its management, or by a new range of treatments which are less problematical. That Prozac, claimed to be one of the latter, has raised a new set of ethical problems should, however, alert us. Good science is likely to be ethical, by definition, but though morality will also demand good research and a clear knowledge base, the focus of its concerns are elsewhere. The concerns of ethics are, broadly, to answer the question: what is right and what is good? An ethical question is not 'is it *correct* that Happilene dispels depression better than the usual medical treatment?' but 'is it *right* that it does so, in the broadest terms?' Ethics are concerned particularly with issues of conduct or character, with values and veracity, with rights and respect. It may be that the human costs of Happilene are too high, that it cures depression by erasing other key positive features of human life such as, say, motivation or inquisitiveness, or that the physical costs cannot be borne by existing resources. Ethics presents therefore a series of challenges to our thinking which may initially make the matter more problematic, but which are necessary if we are to progress to something clearer and better.

THE CHALLENGE OF REALITY

A primitive but insistent challenge is that, in spite of the optimistic tone of health policy makers, there is a Murphy's Law loose in the universe, particularly neatly summed up by the military: 'if things can go wrong, they will. In fact, they already have.' The importance of this is most concisely put by the late Sir Geoffrey Warnock (1992: 449) in *The Object of Morality*, where he also seems to be describing a sort of moral entropy.

> Resources are limited; people are often not rational, they are vulnerable to others, and dependent on others, and yet inevitably often in competition with others; and human sympathies being limited, they may often neither get nor give help that is needed. ... Thus it comes about that there is in what may be called the human predicament a certain 'natural' tendency for things to go very badly.

He might almost have been writing about depressed people, or depression as a medical entity. No one who has lived with a depressed person can fail to feel the resonance of 'human sympathies being limited'. It's not what a carer would *want* to do. Somehow the weakness of the flesh and the spirit combine to make it very hard to continue to care at length with sympathy and understanding for someone who is depressed. Perhaps this is one explanation for our GP failure to diagnose depression in the short run: that we may be too tired, or worn out, or depressed as doctors ourselves to allow ourselves to recognize yet another unhappy person. It's easier to check the haemoglobin and see them again in two weeks. It will probably be all right till then.

But in opposition to this he poses the 'general object' of morality: to make our contribution to the improvement (or non-deterioration) of the human predicament 'primarily and essentially by seeking to countervail "limited sympathies" and their potentially most damaging effects' (Warnock, 1992: 449). However simple this may seem, it is clearly neither easy nor superficial, but particularly liable to be forgotten in the current climate of limiting access to health care in the name of balancing budgets. It would be all too easy, in the infelicitous American insurance phrase, to say 'no dental, no mental' in health care funding. However good it may be 'to sharpen the concept of health' in order to know on what we should be spending our money, as one recent British health secretary said, the Warnock statement should remind us both that medicine is at base a moral not a scientific or purely administrative exercise, and that it would be hard, if not impossible, to undertake this work by making artificial and inhuman distinctions between the mind and the body. *How* we may respond to and treat depression is a question for regular and constant assessment: but that we *should* do so is not open for debate. The Warnockian reality is both in the pessimism of the assessment, and the moral requirement of our response.

THE CHALLENGE OF UNSILENCING

If there is such a thing as moral progress, it is found not just in responding to the range and assessment of the human predicament, but in extending that range by constant review. We should use our understanding of ourselves, as well as our contact with others, to question, for instance, whether it really is good enough to accept that members of a certain ethnic group cannot say they are depressed, or that children cope 'well' with certain experiences. If the challenge of reality is to accept without avoidance that we have a duty to respond to suffering of whatever kind we see, so the challenge of unsilencing is to improve the human predicament by giving the silent a voice. To do this may be to accept that, although previous generations may not have thought of a certain behaviour as wrong or inadequate, attitudes need to change – the moral space may need to be enlarged. Moral progress, as Rorty has remarked, 'depends on expanding this space'. Using feminism as the starting point and exemplar, he suggests: 'Only if somebody has a dream, and a voice to describe that dream, does what looked like nature begin to look like culture, what looked like fate begin to look like a moral abomination' (Rorty, 1995: 126). New descriptions and language may be needed to help this new voice to speak.

This may be just a question of finding how to express something in a language. We are now listening more carefully to the communication of depression at extremes of age. Just as our definition of low mood includes retarded thought and behaviour, reduced energy and feelings of worthlessness, so even the normally articulate may be unable to make themselves heard. But in a deeper way there is a second set of challenges; to enlarge the moral space surrounding our concept of suffering. Taylor has helpfully pointed out that suffering has become a modern obsession (Taylor, 1989). We don't want people to die, and doctors are our agents in this, yes, but we also do not think that anyone, animals included, should suffer. Just as Adam Smith described poverty as lack of those things which are available to other fellow citizens, so we could define suffering as having a similarly constant moving edge. We no longer expect women to give birth in pain. We also have begun to move the boundary of pain away from the purely physical. No pharmacologist could uphold a narrowly physical view of pain control – and Fulford, we remember, has clarified the primacy of the mind in assessment of symptoms – but the old view saw mental suffering as distinct from pain. We are becoming less clear about that distinction, and it may be that the two forms of suffering should be seen as a continuum, rather than in separate compartments. Distress, and the depression that follows it so often, are a form of pain which we are less and less inclined to take for granted or allow to remain unexplained.

One of humanity's most powerful ways of dealing with a negative experience is to talk about it, from the creation of myth to autobiographical writing. It seems like a very physical process, to 'get something off your chest'. Brian Keenan, beginning his account of his terrible ordeal as a hostage in Beirut for nearly five years, quotes D.H. Lawrence as saying that 'writers throw up their sickness in books' (Keenan, 1992). Is it a moral requirement for us to ensure that people who have suffered and are depressed can tell about their suffering, as well as be made better by medication? Certainly the suffering of loneliness, or of not being heard, is seen by many as being acute. For Primo Levi, dreaming in Auschwitz, not being listened to in his sleep removed the last vestiges of hope from a nightmare experience (Levi, 1979). Perhaps one of the lessons learned world wide from the death of Diana, Princess of Wales was that someone who appears to be paying real attention to suffering, at whatever distance, is of huge value to people otherwise trapped between remote and soulless inhumanities, whether in a state system or a market. Modern communications may increase the capacity for contact, but may also increase the potential for crushing aloneness if no one appears to be listening. Researchers currently are tying themselves in knots to discover what is so good about counselling, and whether there is real evidence that it 'works'. People's need to be heard, and the moral imperative behind it, may simply make some of these enquiries non-questions. But how can we examine these different imperatives?

THE CHALLENGE OF CURRENT FRAMEWORKS IN MEDICAL ETHICS

The framework I have used in general practice over the last few years may offer a set of methods (Higgs, 1997). When a person presents to a professional, he or she places himself or herself in a (health care) *system* – with certain regulations – and in a *relationship*. Both have moral constraints and these can be seen looking forward, in *outcomes* or *consequences*, and backwards, as it were, in *duties*. Broadly speaking, these describe the two directions of flow of much mainstream ethical thinking. But the distinction between them may not hold in the clinical encounter, where both may need to be considered and the answers may conflict. Raanan Gillon has been the main proponent in the UK of the system most widely accepted and used: the *four principles* of *respect for autonomy, beneficence, minimizing harm* and *justice* (or fairness) (Gillon, 1994). These general moral principles enable us to begin to weigh up the different aspects of a problem, and each principle (and issue) may have particular *scope*. This excellent currency may still not be detailed enough for all the particular and complex issues of general practice. The principles are necessary, but may not be sufficient, for our task here.

I have suggested three additional approaches. The first considers, within the system and the relationship, particular *roles* and *responsibilities*. The classic situation is the request for life assurance information, as mentioned earlier, where the GP is no longer working solely or even mainly for her patient, and yet this is often not clear to the patient or the doctor herself.

Each role, whether friend, researcher, student teacher, employer or whatever, may have different and sometimes conflicting responsibilities. For instance, the colleague who has just lost a baby and is dealing harshly and apparently insensitively with mothers at the baby clinic needs not only sympathy and understanding: as an employer or a manager of health care, the GP may have additional and overriding responsibilities. These may be linked to the second approach, through the *values* we promote in the service and individual *virtues* or aspects of character. The question here is not so much 'what should a good doctor (or patient) *do*?' as 'what *is* a good doctor (or patient)?' But we still have no direct way of weighing these values against each other any more than we have with the four principles above. The discussion needs to take into account the *perspectives* and *purposes* of all the different actors or potential actors in the drama in order to be in any sense a rounded ethical assessment. Although this may appear to be a tall order of skyscraper proportions, in reality it is in human scale and within our everyday compass. That professionals do this when they're on form, involved in their work and listening well to clients, should not blind us to the need to 'disaggregate' the judgements from the actions in order to understand them, justify them if contentious and learn from the processes. This should help when tiredness, lack of natural sympathy and shortage of time mean that good judgement is at risk. It is likely that many patients will have started the process before coming to the surgery. Gilligan (1982) describes American women in just such a frame when making decisions about abortion. In many consultations, rushed and inadequate as they may be, the participants show the elements of this at work when considering the best way forward. 'Won't these antidepressants make me too sleepy to hear my baby?', 'If I go on like this my work and family will suffer', 'I'm really sorry to come on Saturday, I know it's not an emergency, but I don't think I can go on.' The balancing of harms is now not a theoretical exercise but deeply personal and completely contextualized. The professional problem is both to see the depth and the meaning, and to help someone blinded by low mood to find a positive way out. The principles are there, but applied to a role in practice, and measured out in context, acknowledging individual views and perspectives.

THE CHALLENGE OF DIFFERENT DISCOURSES

The players in a clinical encounter may be seen in more representative mode, as 'patient', 'doctor', 'relative', 'counsellor' and so on, as if we were writing a medical morality play. Although individual perspectives are vital in context, the way in which they describe their feelings and thoughts might well depend on their background and training, and the way they 'saw' depression. We have assumed up to a point the importance of a medical discourse on mental illness: that it is indeed a doctor's business, that it is helpfully seen as an illness, or even as a disease which can be treated, that it may be cured and prevented, and so on; that person is a patient who, as the word implies, suffers and that this status is appropriate. All that may appear straightforward. In fact, it is far from unproblematic. The challenge is that not everyone sees it this way: in fact, some who have been through 'the system' adamantly refuse to see it this way ever again.

One of the challenges to the medical discourse comes from those who have been suffering from mental illness and count themselves as 'survivors'. The shock to the medic on such an otherwise welcome meeting is to discover that the survivor considers himself or herself to have survived not the illness, but the treatment: that it is the responses of health service personnel, and not the experiences of the condition, which have provided the greatest threat to health or happiness and to any sense of integrity and meaning. Such a response is more often seen in someone after an experience of psychosis, of madness rather than sadness, but where the depression has been severe or the experience extreme, and where the treatments have been particularly difficult, similar views may be encountered. The practical problem may be that, for the medical person meeting a survivor, during a period where the survivor is 'well' and the discussion theoretical, the interchange may be tough but fruitful; whereas when an 'illness' has struck again it may preclude any co-operation, and the doctor and potential patient are from the beginning on different sides of a battle line:

> 'My worst failure was, I think, when this isolated 35-year-old man became suicidal, and I had to admit him to a psychiatric ward under section. My mistake was perhaps to make no contact when he was an inpatient. Certainly later when I visited the ward for a different reason I saw what a cuckoo's nest it really was – you had to be mad to survive it intact, to be sure. Anyway, when he was discharged he decided, though apparently better, to withdraw from any medical contact at all. Though officially on our list, he wouldn't reply to letters, wouldn't talk to me on the phone, and wouldn't let me past the front door. He's not taking medication now, and as he has been diagnosed as having a bipolar condition I'm just sitting here biting my nails.'
>
> (GP in a group discussing successes and failures in treatment of depression)

This person may simply be reacting to a bad experience, but this account suggests that it is something more. The former patient has, in spite of the experience of a severe depression, rejected the medical model altogether.

Under normal circumstances a person now has the choice as to whether to be a patient or not. Someone with diabetes mellitus may simply choose to take his chances rather than the treatment: the law backs ethics in the UK in providing no way that a doctor may properly take action without consent, unless risking a charge of assault. Severe mental conditions are, strangely, an exception, perhaps because of the danger to public rather than purely private health. But even when there is no danger of madness or mayhem, this different approach appears to sanction doctors taking a much less 'autonomy-centred' view of treatment and treatment choices than they might do in physical illness.

Another area in this disputed field is antidepressant medicine, which often has unpleasant side effects, especially at the doses considered to be effective. Here a professional in primary care can feel torn, knowing all too well both the unpleasantness of the effects and the dangers of inadequate treatment. However, two other discourses come to mind to complicate things further: that of the psychotherapist and that of the sociologist. For effective therapy to start, many therapists would see an attitude of depression to be, as it were, a starting gate. 'Breakdown' can provide the way for 'breakthrough', where a defended and hitherto functioning person meets the long-term intrapsychic effects of ignoring part of his or her makeup – but at a price. Depression may be distressing in the extreme but in this way of thinking it is the beginning of the way back, not something just to be blotted out or 'cured'. This attitude is not alien to other thinking in mainstream medical mental health care. For instance, all would agree that addicted individuals, especially alcoholics, might have to hit rock bottom before reality dawns and shows them the road to recovery. In depression, few psychotherapists would work thus with the suicidal, but depression is seldom thought of as a possible 'good' in most psychiatric clinics. There is also the philosophical challenge that it is being *happy* in some situations which would be pathological (Bentall, 1992). Such radical ideas underline the ontological difficulty about depression. Clearly in some situations it may be a life-saver, rather than the reverse. An evolutionary thinker might suggest that having a low mood or energy level is a way in which an animal, human or otherwise, is able to survive defeat or dominance, by reducing struggle and aggression and focusing on the goal of 'just getting by'. The philosophical gloss to this would be to see low mood as in some senses more in the *value* than the *fact* camp: though depression could be objectively determined, its meaning or value would determine whether it were best seen as pathology, as potential, as personality or as part of the normal pattern of life.

These ideas are helpful in general practice, but the sociological discourse may be even more so. Depression in primary care so often follows some unpleasant (to the patient) life event or occurrence. The link is *loss*: the person loses something or someone of value, or fails to meet a social goal. Studies of this process are most advanced in respect of women, and the key exponent is Brown (1996). His instrument (the Life Events and Difficulties Schedule) 'has been good enough to establish that certain kinds of nasty event do occur quite soon before onset in the majority of depressive disorders and that they are of etiological significance' (1996: 37). To loss he adds the *challenge to identity* – that a role or cherished idea about the individual or someone near to the individual may be at risk or be destroyed. His latest work links these ideas to humiliation, entrapment, powerlessness and defeat. Sometimes these ideas can only be understood by entering the person's frame of reference. It is likely that this etiology is very largely the one workers are used to in primary care, while the less common 'endogenous' or unprovoked depression is more commonly encountered in specialist psychiatry.

THE CHALLENGE OF COMMON SENSE

Unpopular as the concept of common sense is with academic thinkers, there is an everyday demotic discourse to be found which is surprisingly decisive. People who are depressed in a way we cannot understand, endogenous severe depressives, should be treated as ill, even to the point where if they are making really understandable threats to their own lives our duty to help or prevent harm trumps respect for their autonomy, at least for the time being. The common sense argument would always want to give someone who is suicidal a second chance. Doctors in their covenant with society would find it hard to escape this requirement. But when the outlook really *is* bleak, as in desperate unremitting suffering both mental and physical, the common voice suggests that death may not be the worst thing: it is possible to be trapped in a terrible life (Higgs, 1977). (This view would not be severe on the doctor who, in defiance of the law, actively aided such a 'rational' suicide.) What is terrible, in this view, is being treated without being listened to, being, as one of my own patients once said, 'vetted rather than doctored' – reduced, as she explained when apologising for her unusual use of English, to an animal to be medicated rather than a person to be responded to, who wants to understand and be understood, who needs events to give meaning in an apparently meaningless landscape.

THE CHALLENGE OF THE DOCTOR'S OWN PERSON

There may be a range of reasons why professionals in primary care do not respond to depression. There may be too much of it about, and a feeling that so little can be done to help some who live in desperate and insoluble situations. Helping people is very tiring. Professionals too have autonomy and can (and probably should) choose to preserve themselves rather than go under. But why some doctors are so deaf to depression remains a conundrum, backlit by a new understanding that many in practice are sufficiently depressed to be cases themselves. There is no space to explore this here beyond saying that the motivation to medicine may carry a specific risk to depression, and that a doctor has a duty to look to her own mental health, just as much as to keep up to date (Higgs, 1994). A wounded healer whose wound stinks so much that no one can come near is no healer at all.

A WAY FORWARD

These challenges are satisfying in that they do provide some useful outcomes and a map, if not precise route directions, for a way forward. Safety and saving lives are, as always, key imperatives, but responding to the suffering of depression, loneliness and despair is increasingly laid at a doctor's door. Effective treatment will not just entail getting the dose of medication right. If the evidence base is the evidence of need as well as outcome, people also are expressing the need to be listened to. For the majority of depressed people seen in primary care, there is a story to be heard, which may take time, which may need the help of others. The responsibility is laid on professionals in this field to see detecting and responding as their business, intervening too where necessary. But it is also a responsibility to ensure that there is a service, and that the service (including themselves) is fit to deal with depressed people of all sorts, at a time and in a way in which these people need help. Difficult cases may be exceptions which prove (i.e. *test*) the rule, rather than creating a climate of rule-breaking. Yet every judgement is in context and needs to be justified by good moral thinking. Taking time out to reflect on our practice, to take our bearings, to review the map and our position is not an optional extra. It requires continual movement between theory and practice, or between evidence-based medicine and the minute everyday particulars of responding as well as possible to this distressed person today in this surgery.

KEY POINTS

- It is likely that every judgement in this field has a moral component
- Doctors are required to pay attention as well as offer access, to listen as well as act
- The boundary of the ethical in this area is on the move
- Different views of depression and mental health may offer a properly rounded assessment in primary care

REFERENCES

Bebbington, P., Hurry, J., Tennant, C., Sturt, E. and Wing, J. (1981) 'Epidemiology of Mental Disorders in Camberwell', *Psychological Medicine*, 11: 561–81.

Bentall, R.P. (1992) 'A proposal to classify happiness as a psychiatric disorder', *Journal of Medical Ethics*, 18: 94–8.

Brown, G.W. (1996) 'Life events, loss and depressive disorders', in T. Heller, J. Reynolds, R. Gomm, R. Muston and S. Pattison (eds) *Mental Health Matters*, London: Open University Press.

Freeling, P. and Tylee, A. (1992) 'Depression in general practice', in E.S. Paykel (ed.) *Handbook of Affective Disorders* (2nd edn), Edinburgh: Churchill Livingstone.

Freeling, P., Rao, B.M., Paykel, E.S., Sireling, L.I. and Burton, R.H. (1985) 'Unrecognised depression in general practice', *British Medical Journal*, 290:1180–3.

Fulford, K.W.M. (1989) *Moral Theory and Medical Practice*, Cambridge: Cambridge University Press.

Gillon, R. (ed.) (1994) *Principles of Health Care Ethics*, Chichester: Wiley.

Gilligan, C. (1982) *In a Different Voice*, Cambridge, Mass.: Harvard University Press.

Goldstein, R.B., Black, D.W., Nasrallah, A. and Winokur, G. (1991) 'The Prediction of Suicide', *Arch General Psychiatry*, 48: 418–22.

Higgs, R. (1977) 'Death My Only Love'. *Journal of Medical Ethics*, 3: 93–7.

Higgs, R. (1994) 'Doctors in crisis: creating a strategy for mental health in health care work', *Journal of the Royal College of Physicians of London*, 28: 538–40.

Higgs, R. (1997) 'Shaping our ends: the ethics of respect in a well-led NHS'. *British Journal of General Practice*, 47: 245–9.

Keenan, B. (1992) *An Evil Cradling*, London: Hutchinson.
Levi, P. (1979) *If This is a Man*, London: Penguin.
Mann, A. (1992) 'Depression and anxiety in primary care: the epidemiological evidence', in R. Jenkins, J. Newton and R. Young (eds) *The Prevention of Depression and Anxiety*. London: HMSO.
Rorty, R. (1995) 'Feminism and pragmatism' in: R. Goodman (ed.) *Pragmatism: A Contemporary Reader*, New York: Routledge.
Rutz, W., Carlsson, P., von Knorring, L. and Walinder, J. (1992) 'Cost benefit analysis of an educational program for general practitioners by the Swedish Committee for the Prevention and Treatment of Depression', *Acta Psychiatry Scandinavia*, 85: 457–64.
Scott, J., Eccleston, D. and Boys, R. (1992) 'Can we predict the persistence of depression?', *British Journal of Psychiatry*, 161: 633–7.
Taylor, C. (1989) *Sources of the Self: The Making of the Modern Identity*, Cambridge: Cambridge University Press.
Warnock, G.J. (1992) 'The object of morality', in A.J. Ayer and J. O'Grady (eds) *A Dictionary of Philosophical Quotations*, Oxford: Blackwell.
Wilber, J.A. and Barrow, J.G. (1972) 'Hypertension – a community problem', *American Journal of Medicine*, 52: 653–63.
Williams, P. and Clare, A. (1979) *Psychological Disorders in General Practice*, London: Academic Press.

Chapter 9

Advance directives

Angus Dawson

INTRODUCTION

Advance directives are statements by competent patients about what medical treatment they want or do not want if at some point in the future they become incompetent. Advance directives are presently most often invoked when talking about medical care at the end of life (hence their common name, 'living wills'), but they are increasingly suggested as a way of contributing towards ethical practice in other areas of health care. It is imperative that everyone working in health care today has a clear idea of the legal and ethical issues that surround the issue of advance directives as their use is only likely to increase in the future.

There are a number of reasons why directives are becoming increasingly popular. The first are the general social and political changes which have occurred in the nature of the professional–patient relationship, with a growing dissatisfaction with the perceived paternalism of traditional health care and a movement towards a new emphasis upon patient autonomy (President's Commission, 1982; Gillon, 1986). This change in attitude is perhaps best illustrated by the increasing acceptance of the need to gain the informed consent of a patient prior to any health care intervention. An 'informed consent' is the end product of a free decision by a competent patient about their own treatment, based upon an understanding of information about the nature of the procedure, the intended outcome, possible risks and side-effects and possible alternatives (Faden and Beauchamp, 1986; Appelbaum *et al.*, 1987). The same motivation can be seen behind the drive to produce advance directives. The only difference is that directives are attempts by a presently competent individual to control future, rather than contemporaneous decisions about their health care. The President's Commission (1983), for example, held that advance directives should be encouraged because they are the best way of maximizing the incompetent patient's involvement in decision making about their own treatment. Many of the professional bodies in the UK agree, and have advocated support for advance directives (BMA, 1993, 1995).[1] When patients are asked for their views on directives, they tend to be favourable (Emanuel *et al.*, 1991a; Gamble *et al.*, 1991). There has been little investigation into patient attitudes towards directives in the UK, but where there has, the same enthusiasm is apparent.[2]

The second, related influence is the public's concern about the nature of the changes in medicine in recent years. There is increasing anxiety that the development of, for example, modern resuscitation techniques, life-support technology and new drugs all mean that an individual's death may be delayed beyond the point at which it would otherwise have occurred. There is also a common perception that the use of medical technology itself may be the cause of undesirable consequences; for example, leading to conditions such as persistent vegetative state (PVS). These attitudes have been partly formed and reinforced by media reactions to high profile legal cases, which illustrate some of these points.[3] It is thought that advance directives provide a way for a patient to seek to prevent themselves from becoming such a victim.

A third, and growing, influence has been the development of various interest groups with a keen interest in the issue of advance directives. Perhaps most media attention is fixed on various pro-euthanasia groups who see advance directives as being within their general remit.[4] However, there are other groups that have led the debate in the UK. For example, one of the most thorough early treatments of the issue in this country was the booklet produced by Age Concern and the Centre of Medical Law and Ethics at King's College London (1988); and perhaps one of the most active groups in campaigning for the introduction and validity of directives has been the Terrence Higgins Trust, which has published draft directives and conducted surveys of patient and health care workers' attitudes towards directives (Schlyter, 1992). This lead might be because it is those with their minds focused upon death who are most likely to formulate a directive, and because the majority of sufferers from HIV and AIDS are young, articulate and determined to fight for their rights. Advance directives provide a clear way of attempting to secure them.

Advance directives originated as written documents that established which possible medical interventions an individual wished to refuse when they entered the last stages of a terminal illness. However, the concept of a directive has now broadened beyond this, so the first part of this chapter will explore a number of issues relating to the nature of directives, including discussion of the form of the directive, the different types of option that are available, the different types of situation where they may be used and whether there may be any limits placed on the type of requests that could be made.

DIFFERENT FORMS OF ADVANCE DIRECTIVES

The first issue to be considered is the form that a directive should take. For example, an advance directive might be either oral or written. In the latter form they draw upon an analogy with testamentary dispositions in that they are written and witnessed documents, and this is why they are popularly termed 'living wills'.[5] Although this type of document is still perhaps the paradigm advance directive, it is no longer the only instance in which a directive can be given and applied. I will therefore use the term advance directive through out this chapter rather then 'living will' to emphasize the range and flexibility of the format. If we think of directives as being instructions to govern health care decision making for the patient if they become incompetent, then it is clear that such instructions could also be given in oral form to the health care staff or to the patient's family or friends. This means that the idea of an advance directive can range, in practice, from a single whispered sentence to a substantial multi-page signed and witnessed written document. The correct place of oral wishes within the care of the incompetent is unclear, but they have been accepted as binding by the courts.[6] The chief advantage of a written document is an evidential one, in that it is less likely to be open to dispute. So, just as there are many different types of directive, so there may be different degrees of willingness to follow and enforce them.

THE NATURE OF REQUESTS MADE IN ADVANCE DIRECTIVES

Whatever formal requirements are considered necessary for validity, the next issue to consider is the nature of the requests that can be made. Some directives provide detailed statements on the types of treatment that are requested or refused; others seek to appoint a trusted 'proxy' or 'substitute' decision maker, someone to make decisions on the patient's behalf; other directives seek to combine these two approaches, allowing the proxy to play a role as interpreter of the statements, where necessary.[7] What are the advantages and disadvantages of each of these options?

Interpretation of written instructions

Eisendrath and Jonsen (1983) argue that directives help medical staff and the patient's family with decision making about the patient's treatment. However, if instruction directives are to be useful they need to overcome a number of possible problems. For example, the requests that they state might be either too specific or not specific enough. A good illustration of this problem is the instruction directive called a 'Medical Directive' formulated by Emanuel and Emanuel (1989). This directive is in the form of a detailed document which specifies exactly what treatment an individual would want in a list of full treatment scenarios. However, as Erin and Harris (1994) suggest, this type of directive may be too detailed and prove too cumbersome to use. Paradoxically, the more detailed a directive, the more likely it is to fail to apply to the particular situation required as it is impossible for a single directive to cover every possible eventuality. If the particular situation is not covered, are the medical staff to resort to a best interests test or try and 'apply' another part of the directive to that situation?

An alternative solution would be to try and formulate the original directive in as broad a way as possible so that this situation doesn't arise. Some commentators have argued that such a directive would seek to outline the patient's general attitudes and views towards such things as different types of treatment and incompetence itself, so that their values could then be applied to any individual situation that arises. Such directives are called 'General Values Directives' (Gibson and Nathanson, 1990; Doukas and McCullough, 1991). However, this lack of any detailed instructions can also lead to problems in that by definition the directive will need to be applied to the specific situation, and this opens up the possibility of differing interpretations of what a patient might want in a particular situation.

This problem is made even more difficult if the language used in the instruction directive is vague. This was certainly a fault with many early directives. For example, the 'living will' proposed by Modell (1974) says that there should be no treatment 'of any sort' if there is a decline in mental capacity. Is a reader of this directive always to interpret this literally? For example, it might well be possible to give a treatment that reverses that decline; if one were available, should this not be given? Brock (1991) makes a similar point in his discussion of which situations might require a directive to be overridden. He gives the example of a directive instructing that CPR (Cardiopulmonary resuscitation) should not be given. Do we need to be clearer about a patient's intentions behind this type of instruction? The patient might only mean that CPR should be withheld when her overall medical condition is poor and not in situations where CPR could almost certainly restore her to her previous lifestyle. Should an interpreter of the directive follow the letter of the instructions, or attempt to carry out an interpretation based upon the supposed intentions of the patient?[8]

Other directives revolve around particular words or phrases that are vague and the interpretation of them is likely to be essential to deciding what to do. Examples of the type of words that might present difficulties are those often used to describe unwanted treatments, such as 'extraordinary', 'heroic' and 'futile' (Wolf *et al.*, 1991); or interpreting phrases such as a wish 'not to be a burden' (Pellegrino and Thomasma, 1988). Attempts have been made to clarify such phrases, but suggestions such as that of Schneiderman *et al.*, 1990 that 'futile' treatment can be defined as medical treatment that has failed to work for the last 100 times that it has been used seem rather arbitrary. To confirm that such issues to do with the problem of interpretation are not merely academic, it is worth noting the real life experiences of doctors such as Rosner (1994) and Taranta (1994) that confirm the difficulty that such vague language in directives presents in practice.

A more devastating objection to this type of directive arises from empirical evidence which questions the degree to which an advance directive can ever capture what the author would want to happen when it comes down to the actual application of the directive. For example, it is unclear whether the views outlined in an advance directive are really the settled views of the author because there is much evidence that patients are likely to change their minds about what they want (Loewy, 1988; Silverstein *et al.*, 1991; Everhart and Perlman, 1990; Emanuel *et al.*, 1991b). Even if an advance directive contains a fair summary of an individual's views, it is not clear that patients always mean them to be followed. For example, one study (Sehgal *et al.*, 1992) even suggests that those who complete directives do not necessarily want their future treatment to be determined by those documents! The message seems to be that they want to allow the possibility of some sort of 'leeway' in interpretation and application.

It has been argued by some that these types of objections to instruction directives can be overcome as long as a couple of rules are followed. For example, the BMA (1993, 1995) argue that directives are best formulated by patients through a process of dialogue with their doctors so that the directive corresponds to current medical thinking. Their advice is to keep the document as simple and as general as possible. It is hoped that this will allow the production of realistic directives that avoid the kind of ambiguities that have been discussed above. Whether this is possible remains to be seen. However, it should not be assumed that these problems can necessarily be overcome by simply appointing a substitute decision maker through a proxy directive, as this raises a new set of possible problems.

Problems with proxies

A proxy directive is one way of attempting to allow decision making about treatment decisions to be influenced by the patient's own views through a substitute who is chosen by the patient to make such decisions on their behalf (Juengst and Weil, 1989). The advantage of a proxy is that they can respond to the particularities of the patient's actual circumstances and make a decision in response to them. The proxy can be informed at the time of all the aspects necessary to make an informed consent, such as the risks and benefits of treatment and the availability of any possible alternative treatments. Appointing a proxy means that the issues around ambiguity and problems of interpretation are less likely to arise because the proxy can also be questioned about the views that they put forward.

There are two different types of judgement that might be used as a basis for a proxy's decision making. A proxy might produce a judgement about what they believe the *patient would want*, based upon their knowledge of the patient's views and values. This is called a 'substituted judgement'. An alternative type of judgement could be delivered by a proxy given the power by the patient's directive to make decisions about the patient's medical treatment on the basis of what the *proxy believes* is in the patient's best interests; and therefore this can be called a 'best interests' test.

Most proxies are of the substituted judgement form, as this seems to be the best way of involving the individual patient's own views most directly in the decision-making process. However, there are a number of possible problems with such directives. For example, it might be hard to determine whether the proxy is representing the true views of the patient rather than their own (assuming there is a difference). Is there any way of instituting a check on such decisions? Should it be possible to overrule such judgements if it is thought that a proxy is overstepping or abusing their position? To what extent is it actually possible for one individual to represent another's views independently of their own? Emanuel and Emanuel (1992: 2068) argue that proxy decisions require 'huge imaginative effort', as well as the ability to neutralize the proxy's own bias, prejudices and psychological agenda. This is perhaps a special problem where possible conflicts of interest might emerge (La Puma and Schiedermayer, 1991).

Even if these factors to do with one individual 'representing' another could be overcome, there are further possible problems. For example, is such a judgement more than an 'informed' guess? Empirical studies that have looked at the adequacy of decisions made by proxies seem to produce disturbing results for the supporters of this form of directives (Emanuel and Emanuel, 1992). This research suggests that proxies fail to adequately ascertain the patient's wishes about health care scenarios, even about their attitudes towards such common events as CPR;[9] that proxies tend to assess quality of life judgements differently from the patients themselves;[10] and that proxies often produce different answers about appropriate treatment in response to treatment scenarios from those produced by the patients themselves.[11] Even though Lynn (1992) rightly argues for caution in interpreting such empirical studies (a warning that Emanuel and Emanuel make themselves (1992)), it is hard to conclude anything but that, at the very least, more thought needs to be given to how this form of proxy decision making can better achieve its aims. Given the scale of these problems, the possibility should remain open that these inadequacies are fundamental and cannot be overcome.

The 'substituted judgement' form of proxy directives gain their popularity from the idea that they allow a greater expression of an individual's own views and feelings. However, it is possible to question this through a consideration of the conceptual objection put forward by Gutheil and Appelbaum (1983), who argue that such judgements allegedly made on the basis of a substituted judgement are really only disguised forms of a best interests test applied to particular examples. Such a test is, of course, the basis of the second form of proxy directive. This type of directive consists of the proxy making a decision, on behalf of the patient, based upon what the proxy holds to be the treatment in that patient's 'best interest'. However, if this is to be the basis of the decision to be made on behalf of the patient, it is worth asking why it should be made by the proxy rather than by anyone else? If 'best interests' for an individual are possible to determine (and this is doubted by some), why should others not be better at determining them than the proxy? For example, as we are talking here about medical decision making, might not best interests be better determined by someone who understands all of the medical facts? If medical decisions are to be made for incompetent patients strictly on the basis of a 'best interests' test, then it is hard to see what purpose a directive serves.

A third form of directive, and one that is becoming increasingly popular in the US, is a 'mixed' directive that seeks to combine an instruction directive with the appointment of a proxy. In such cases, the proxy is employed to clear up any ambiguities or problems about the application in the particular situations, but the patient's clear instructions can be used as a guide in decision making. It is thought by their supporters that these 'mixed' directives combine the advantages of and meet the objections to the two previous forms of directives discussed above. However, it is not clear that they can do so; and in fact they might create further problems of their own.

WHEN DO ADVANCE DIRECTIVES COME INTO OPERATION?

A further area where there has been a broadening of the role of directives is over what might be called the 'triggering event'; that is, the point at which they come into operation. This is standardly taken to be the moment at which the patient becomes incompetent or incapacitated. However, it has been suggested by some that an advance directive should only be 'triggered', when a patient is both incompetent *and* has a terminal illness. This type of restriction is still common with many directives formulated following US statutes. However, if directives are enforceable in such situations it is unclear why they should not also govern the treatment of other conditions that may eventually produce incompetence, but are not immediately life-threatening. One example of this might be degenerative conditions such as Huntingdon's disease, Parkinson's disease and dementia. Perhaps this restriction is just a remnant of the origins of directives in treatment decisions at the end of life and will change over time.

If such a restriction is unjustified then it might be possible to allow a role for directives in situations where a patient might not be strictly incompetent, but feels that an expression of their wishes about treatment decisions would be a useful way of bringing them to the attention of those in charge of their care. This type of directive might be used to support treatment decisions in some of the recent problematical cases involving refusals of treatments, such as those of Caesarean sections or blood transfusions on religious grounds.[12] It has been noted by some that birth plans, the written expression of a pregnant woman's wishes about the care and management of her pregnancy and birth, share some of the features of a directive (Sommerville, 1996). A woman may gain comfort from the fact that she has such a document which she can invoke if need be to demonstrate that her wishes are long standing and informed, despite not strictly being a directive because she is not incompetent. In such a situation, the 'triggering event' would not be incompetence, but a request by the patient.

Another area of medical care where advance directives might play a role is in the treatment of those with a mental illness, for example requesting a refusal of consent to psychiatric medication or hospitalization (Brock, 1993). However, there are some, such as the BMA, who are sceptical of this (BMA, 1993, 1995). It is unclear why, if directives are appropriate for a terminal illness, they should not be so for mental illnesses. The supporters of such a view need to be able to distinguish the cases in some way if they hold that there is a difference.[13] If it is 'clinically inappropriate' (BMA, 1993: 162) to respect an advance directive in this situation, and to resort to 'paternalism' or 'best interests', why does this not cast doubt upon the adequacy of other advance directives? If respecting patient autonomy is a justification in one case, why not the other? If anything, the mental illness case could perhaps be seen as more justified because the authors of them are likely to have had previous experience of their illness, and therefore have an insight into the condition that they seek to avoid that many of the people who produce an advance directive for the end of life will never have.

However the role of advance directives develops in the future, the need to be able to clearly distinguish between the competent and the incompetent will remain so that it can be ascertained when a directive comes into force. This means that it is imperative that there is a clear and agreed definition of incompetence, and that there are clear criteria for determining such incompetence. However, the actual process of determining when an individual is incompetent is the subject of much argument.[14] It is apparent that many judgements about patient incompetence or incapacity are still made in an 'intuitive' manner rather than by following any existing guidelines.

LIMITS TO THE TYPES OF REQUESTS MADE IN ADVANCE DIRECTIVES

Are there any limits to the requests that can be made under an advance directive? For example, directives originated largely as a reaction to perceived 'over-treatment' of the terminally ill, and so far, most emphasis has been placed on refusing particular medical treatment, for example resuscitation, technological assistance, antibiotics, nutrition and hydration.[15] However, there is no reason, in principle, why directives cannot be used to request *positive* intervention. An advance directive might be constructed to request every possible treatment with the aim of seeking to prolong life at all costs; or there may be an instruction which specified a positive request for a particular treatment.

This raises the issue whether there are legitimate restrictions upon the types of requests that can be made in a directive. For example, it is presumably forbidden to request illegal acts (e.g. active euthanasia); but it might also be held to be inappropriate to make requests which absorb substantial resources. This, of course, raises the issue of justice and the obligations on one individual to not receive more than their 'fair share' of resources. Perhaps this is one case where there are clear limits to be placed upon an individual's autonomous requests in a directive. If so, there may be clear limits to the positive treatment that might be enforced, even if clearly and autonomously requested. Kapp (1982) argues that this is unfair and that what he terms a 'directive to provide maximum care' should be implemented if a patient has formulated a request in this manner. He argues that this will enhance patient autonomy and will not result in a large increase in the use of resources because, he hypothesizes, few people are likely to want such a directive. However, it should be borne in mind that the UK courts have proved extremely reluctant to enforce any 'right' to resources in the past, and are as unlikely to be as willing to enforce 'positive', as they are 'negative' requests.[16]

A related issue is whether the application of advance directives will enable the redistribution of health care resources from terminal care to other areas of need. Some have claimed that it could be possible to save money here and that this is a further reason to support the widest possible implementation of directives (Thomasma, 1989). It has even been suggested that the US Congress passed the Patient Self-Determination Act, 1990, which links state medical funding to the promotion of advance directives, with the deliberate aim of saving state funding on health care (La Puma *et al.*, 1991). Chambers *et al.* (1994) suggest that the care of individuals without advance directives was three times as expensive during their final illness. However, two other studies contradict this and suggest that advance directives make no difference to the cost of terminal care (Schneiderman *et al.*, 1992; Teno *et al.*, 1994). This is something that could usefully be the subject of further study; though no doubt some would hold that the question of cost should be irrelevant to proper terminal care.

THE LEGAL BACKGROUND TO ADVANCE DIRECTIVES

The legal position regarding advance directives in the UK is in the process of development. Even though there have been a number of cases which have discussed some of the different types of request that might be part of a directive, there has as yet been no definitive case that has reviewed all of the issues and clearly outlined when a directive will be enforced and when it will not. It would be useful to have these issues clarified by the courts as soon as possible, but, until they are, any discussion must be based upon the application of general legal principles and related cases. Based upon this evidence we can state that it is certainly the case that some sorts of advance directives are legally valid and will therefore be enforced by the courts in the UK.

So how does the law stand at the moment? It is a general legal principle that there can be no medical treatment without a genuine consent.[17] It does not matter whether the decision made is unusual, or even considered irrational, as long as the patient is competent.[18] It would therefore seem natural to extend these principles to advance directives and argue that they are a way of ensuring continued respect for the choices an individual has made even after they have become incompetent. The central problem in interpreting the relevant law is clearly stating which types of requests will be enforced. Perhaps the best summary of the current legal position is provided by the Law Commission (1995), where the writers distinguish an 'anticipatory decision' from the expression of 'wishes', 'views' or 'feelings'. The latter would only be treated as advisory and therefore only be one of many things to be taken into account in making a clinical judgement. The former, however, would be binding as long as it can be shown to apply to the particular facts of the situation and was made in contemplation of those facts. This means that the courts are likely to adopt a very narrow reading of any advance statement, especially if following it would bring about the death of an individual.

This view derives from the case of *Re T* (1992) where a woman in late pregnancy was advised to have a Caesarean section after a road accident. She made a statement that she wished to refuse blood products. She was advised that it was unlikely that they would be necessary in the circumstances. Her condition deteriorated to the extent that her life was held to be in danger. Members of her family applied to the courts to seek agreement to the blood transfusion which it was thought to be necessary to save her life. It was held by the court that her refusal of blood products was invalid in the circumstances because it was not made in contemplation of the life-threatening circumstances that later came about.[19] The 'directive' in this case was oral and it was not considered whether it would make any difference if the directive had been written or had been produced before there was any call for medical treatment (as in the Canadian case of *Malette v Shulman* (1990)). It might also be significant that there was evidence that her refusal was not as the result of a deep personal commitment, as she was not a practising Jehovah's Witness, and may have been unduly influenced by her mother, who was.

Another legal case that considered some of the related legal issues was *Re C* (1994). In this case, a paranoid schizophrenic sought an injunction to prevent his gangrenous leg being amputated in the future. Some of the medical team caring for him believed that he might die if an amputation was not performed. The judge held that he was competent enough to make this decision and that he understood the consequences of such a refusal. However, it should be noted that this case followed the directions laid down in *Re T*, and that this was a very clear refusal of a particular treatment by an informed and competent individual. It is unclear how these cases relate to the application of the full written and witnessed instruction directives discussed above. There would appear to be a paradox at the heart of the current legal position towards directives in that it may be important to formulate the directive before a subsequent illness so that the competence of the patient cannot be questioned. However, the more the directive is formulated prior to its intended use, the less likely it is to be relevant to that particular treatment, and thereby less likely to be legally enforceable!

Another important limitation of the legal attitude to advance directives in England and Wales is that there is no provision in law for proxy decision making in health care.[20] Indeed, it is a general principle of law that no person can consent for another (*Re F* (1990)). This is one important difference from the US, where proxy and substituted judgements have been a popular way of making health care decisions for the incompetent. Indeed, it was the inadequacies in the law, uncovered by *Re F*, and the discussion that it created, that led to the setting up of the Law Commission investigation, that eventually produced the document *Mental Incapacity* (1995). Therefore, as the legal position in England and Wales stands, only the statement form of directives could possibly be enforceable, and as we have seen that opens up the prospect of the courts being filled with arguments about the interpretation of whether or not particular clauses apply to the facts.

Given these limitations, it has been suggested by a number of commentators that the best solution would be parliamentary intervention and new statutory provision (Age Concern/KCL Working Party, 1988; Law Commission, 1995).[21] Unfortunately there has appeared to be a general reluctance amongst politicians to debate anything that might involve discussion of the issue of euthanasia;[22] and there have been many influential opponents of legislation, including the House of Lords Select Committee and the BMA. The latter oppose statutory intervention because they feel it will restrict the future development of flexible directives.[23] This has been the central focus of some opponents of directives, such as Kass (1980), who argues that statutes, court decisions, and guidelines are all unnecessary interferences with the professional judgement of the doctor. It looked, until very recently, as though future legal developments relating to directives would only occur through the development of case law. However, in December 1997, the new Lord Chancellor published a green paper called *Who Decides?: Making Decisions on Behalf of Mentally Incapacitated Adults*, which suggests that legislation is to be introduced, broadly along the lines proposed by the Law Commission.

ADVANCE DIRECTIVES: A ROLE FOR PRIMARY CARE?

Empirical research in the US suggests that the best time to bring up the topic of advance directives with patients may not be in a hospital, but rather in the more relaxed surroundings of the primary care setting.[24] Davidson and Moseley (1989) argue that 'primary care physicians' should take an active role in identifying patients with illnesses where it might be appropriate to formulate a directive and encourage them to do so. This might be one way of ensuring that it is not just the educated and articulate middle classes who formulate directives. There is good evidence that such intervention does increase the rate of drafting directives (Markson *et al.*, 1994). In fact, it is already happening that patients are turning to their GPs for help in formulating their directives.[25] One possibly relevant difference here might be the fact that, in the US, physician care is private, and hence there might be an added incentive to talk to patients at length about their directives. Are busy UK GPs willing to spend anything from 13 to 40 minutes[26] discussing such directives without remuneration?

The BMA suggests that GPs should have a key role in the development of directives because of their existing function as 'gatekeepers' to most NHS services. This means that they are perfectly placed to perform the task, mentioned before, of helping to formulate appropriate and realistic directives. GPs might also be the most appropriate people to keep a copy of a patient's directive. The patient could carry a card stating where it is stored so that, in the event of hospital admission, it can be consulted by those caring for the patient (BMA, 1995: 27). Perhaps, in future, this role of the GP might be strengthened to the extent that it becomes a duty of the GP to bring a directive to the attention of other health care professionals who come to have contact with the patient.

SOME POSSIBLE PROBLEMS WITH ADVANCE DIRECTIVES

In the course of the discussion so far, we have discussed a number of practical problems with advance directives. It might be argued by their supporters that these are all minor problems that can be overcome by, for example, having clear guidelines about implementation. Whether or not this is true, there are a number of more philosophical objections to directives that also need to be answered. Perhaps the most important of these are a group of objections which question the very coherence of advance directives by asking whether they can ever do what they seek to achieve because the link between the previously competent and now incompetent person is broken.

These objections to the very coherence of an advance directive all relate to the philosophical issue of personal identity and what it is to be a unique individual over time.[27] For example, as we have seen, the central reason given to support the idea of directives is that they are held to be the best way of maintaining the patient's autonomous control over their own treatment. However, it might be objected that as the patient is (by *definition*) incompetent, how can *their* autonomy be promoted? Why should an incompetent individual's life be controlled by what they wished for when competent when, by reason of the decline into incompetence, there has been such a significant cognitive change that we might doubt whether they are in any relevant sense the same person? Perhaps in these circumstances it makes no sense to talk of trying to promote such a person's autonomy. Against this sort of claim, it has been argued by some that every individual has their own persisting 'critical interests' (Dworkin, 1993). Once these are expressed by a competent individual, they persist beyond the decline of the individual into incompetence and provide a framework for decision making about their health care treatment. However, it could be counter-argued that this idea creates the thought that there is somehow a homuncular 'real self' that persists and continues to 'govern' or 'bind' the later incompetent self, and that such an idea is obscure, if not incoherent.[28]

The supporters of advance directives should not be quick to dismiss this as 'merely' a philosophical argument, as it can be supported with a number of practical points. The thought that patient wishes might not endure over time has already been alluded to above; but this difficulty cannot just be met by stating that a directive should be reviewed every five years. This is to miss the point of the objection. The idea is rather that the very nature of an advance directive is incoherent because prospective decision making is very different from contemporaneous decision making. This is because you can be fully informed[29] about treatment here and now, but you cannot be informed about your future medical condition, and the different options available to you then. This is because it is both uncertain what medical conditions you might develop in the future and also likely that the writer of an advance directive has no experience of the very states that they wish to avoid.[30] It might be argued that one can only truly have experience of a state when one is in it or has a sound memory of it. There would seem to be a false inference here, from a desire not to be in a particular state to a belief that if one were in that state, life would be unbearable; and this doesn't follow.

The objector to advance directives might argue that instead of an apparently bogus appeal to the previously expressed autonomous wishes of a non-incompetent patient, it is perhaps better to make decisions about health care issues for incompetent patients using a best interests test. This is a more honest position, it might be argued, because it admits to ignorance about what the patient would want in a particular set of circumstances, and that some other criteria rather than a spurious appeal to a patient's autonomous decision making needs to be used. Such a view might be combined with a modest role for advance directives in that, where they are available, or where there is other good evidence of a patient's views, they could be taken into account in a judgement of what the most appropriate treatment might be. In such a situation, the directive would be advisory rather than binding. It might be argued that such a view is the best way of truly respecting patient autonomy; where a patient cannot make decisions about their own care because of incompetence there is no pretence that we can still access a secret well of sustained beliefs.

CONCLUSIONS

The supporters of advance directives often write as though directives are the obvious way to create ethical health care for incompetents. However, as we have seen, there are a number of reasons for caution. There is a strong body of empirical evidence that suggests that there are a number of problems with some of the assumptions lying behind the use of the various forms of advance directives. At the very least, there is a need for much more research on these issues. There are also some strong philosophical arguments against directives, which cannot be ignored and need to be answered. A further reason for caution is that much of our limited experience of directives comes from the US context and, given the differences in our legal and health care systems, there is no reason to think that these findings will translate directly and easily to the UK. It is also important to note that the ethical issues that surround the whole area of the treatment of incompetents cannot simply be solved by invoking the use of directives. It is as well to remember that the majority of the population will never produce a directive, just as they never write a will (Brazier, 1992). One of the aspects of the Law Commission report *Mental Incapacity* (1995) that is to be applauded is that it considered these issues in just such a wider context. It is to be hoped that future discussion of the complex web of issues surrounding medical treatment decisions for incompetents is conducted in a similar sophisticated and subtle manner. Advance directives are, at best, only a partial answer to these difficult legal and ethical issues.

NOTES

1 The BMA booklet (BMA, 1995) was the product of a multi-disciplinary committee set up in response to the House of Lords' Select Committee's Report (1994). *Advance Statements about Medical Treatment* is essentially 'practical' in nature and does not worry about the possible philosophical objections that there might be to directives; but it clearly and concisely sets out many of the relevant issues.

2 See Schlyter (1992) in Kennedy and Grubb (1994: 1340) and the survey from *Yours* magazine, December 1994, reported in Sommerville (1996: 36). However, there is some evidence that this apparent enthusiasm isn't translated into actually drafting directives (Gamble *et al.*, 1991; Sachs *et al.*, 1990; La Puma *et al.*, 1991).

3 Examples might include the US legal cases of, *Quinlan, Re* (1976), *Cruzan v. Missouri Department of Health* (1990) and the UK case of *Airedale NHS Trust v. Bland* (1993).

4 For example, see the evidence of the Voluntary Euthanasia Society to the House of Lords Select Committee (1994).

5 The original idea for a 'living will' was as a direct parallel to a testamentary will; see Kutner (1969).

6 For example, see *Re T* (1992).

7 See Cantor (1993) and King (1996) for the history of these developments in the US legal context.
8 See also Davidson and Moseley (1989) who discuss the interpretation of a similar request for 'no respirator'.
9 Seckler *et al.* (1991); Uhlmann *et al.* (1988); Lo *et al.* (1986); Cohen-Mansfield *et al.* (1991); High (1988); Diamond *et al.* (1989).
10 Epstein (1989); Magaziner *et al.* (1988); Rubenstein (1984).
11 Seckler *et al.* (1991); Tomlinson *et al.* (1990); Zweibel and Cassel (1989); Ouslander *et al.* (1989); Uhlmann *et al.* (1988); Danis *et al.* (1988).
12 For Caesarean sections see *Re S* (1992); and for blood transfusions see *Re T* (1992).
13 The BMA seems to be relying on the idea that the statutory provisions of the Mental Health Act, 1983, will take priority over an advance directive requesting non-treatment in psychiatry (1995: 14). This is almost certainly true, but surely this *legal* fact is not an *ethical* justification for ignoring such a directive.
14 Appelbaum and Grisso (1988); Lo (1990); White (1994); Cutter and Shelp (1991); Brock and Buchanan (1989: Chapter 1); Gunn (1994). For a good general review and a practical guide to the issues see BMA/Law Society (1995).
15 Beauchamp and Childress (1994: 204) comment that some of the US states have refused to recognize a request to terminate nutrition and hydration in their advance directives statutes. However, *Cruzan* (1990); *Jobes, Re* (1987); and, of course, *Bland* (1993) did allow such terminations.
16 See Montgomery (1997: Chapter 3). A recent, and much publicized, case was *R v Cambridge HA ex p. B* (1995). It should also be noted that none of the UK legal cases with any relevance to directives considers positive requests for treatment.
17 See *Re F* (1990).
18 See *Sidaway v Board of Governors Royal Bethlem Hospital* (1985), 666, *per* Lord Templeman.
19 See also the US cases of *In re Estate of Dorone* (1987); *Werth v Taylor* (1991); *In the Matter of Alice Hughes* (1992), cited in Law Commission (1995), where there were similar narrow applications of expressed statements.
20 The Enduring Powers of Attorney Act, 1985, does not apply to medical treatment. However, in Scotland there is some possibility of proxy decision making arising from the powers of a 'tutor dative'. See BMA (1995: 35) and Law Commission (1995: 18–19).
21 Law Commission (1995) contains a careful consideration of many of the relevant issues and includes a draft bill. There was also strong argument from many of the judges involved in the *Bland* case that such questions should be for parliament to settle, rather than being left to develop less formally through the common law.
22 See, for example, the rather half-hearted Government Response to the House of Lords Select Committee Report (1994).
23 Cantor (1993) argues that the US statutes have been a 'major disappointment' for this reason; and Heintz (1988) suggests that ironically legislation can limit patient autonomy.

24 Silverman *et al.* (1994) suggest that there is the scope for a great deal of misunderstanding if directives are discussed as part of admittance to hospital. Patients are generally anxious and suspicious, believing that the issues of directives are only brought up because their health is in fact worse than they are being told. Loewy and Carlson (1994) also argue that discussing directives should be a primary care responsibility.
25 For help on the relevant factors to include in a draft directive see BMA (1995: Part III).
26 Emanuel *et al.* (1991a) and Emanuel (1993).
27 This has been the source of much argument in recent philosophy. See Parfit (1973, 1984); Noonan (1989); Dresser (1989).
28 This is not the place to discuss all the details of such objections and possible replies that might be forthcoming. See Dawson (forthcoming) for more on this.
29 In the sense of 'as much as practically possible'; see Faden and Beauchamp (1986).
30 Ryan (1996) makes a similar point, and reviews a number of empirical studies that suggest that once patients are in a previously undesired state, they have a different perspective from before. He cites three empirical studies to support this: Dillner (1994); Allebeck *et al.* (1989); Brown *et al.* (1986). There is a rather bad tempered response to Ryan's article by Luttrell and Sommerville (1996).

CASES

Airedale NHS Trust v. Bland [1993] 1 All ER 821, HL.
Cruzan v. Missouri Department of Health (1990) 497 US 261, 110 S Ct 2841, US SC.
In re Estate of Dorone (1987) 534 A 2d 452.
In the Matter of Alice Hughes (1992) 611 A 2d 114.
Jobes, Re (1987) 108 NJ 394, NJ SC.
Malette v. Shulman (1990) 67 DLR (4th) 321.
Quinlan, Re (1976) 70 NJ 10, NJ SC.
R v. Cambridge HA, ex p. B [1995] 2 All ER 129, CA.
Re T (adult: refusal of medical treatment) [1992] 4 All ER 649, CA.
Re F (mental patient: sterilisation) [1990] 2 AC 1, HL.
Re C (adult: refusal of medical treatment) [1994] 1 All ER 819.
Re S (adult: refusal of medical treatment) [1992] 4 All ER 671.
Sidaway v. Board of Governors of Royal Bethlem Hospital [1985] 1 All ER 643, HL.
Werth v. Taylor (1991) 190 Mich App 141.

REFERENCES

Age Concern/KCL Working Party (1988) *The Living Will: Consent to Treatment at the End of Life*, London: Arnold.

Allebeck, P. *et al.* (1989) 'Increased suicide rate in cancer patients', *Journal of Clinical Epidemiology*, 42: 611–16.
Appelbaum, P. and Grisso, T. (1988) 'Assessing patients' capacities to consent to treatment', *New England Journal of Medicine*, 319: 1635–8.
Appelbaum, P., Lidz, C. and Meisel, A. (1987) *Informed Consent: Legal Theory and Clinical Practice*, New York: Oxford University Press.
Beauchamp, T. and Childress, J. (1994) *Principles of Biomedical Ethics*, (4th edn), London: Oxford University Press.
Brazier, M. (1992) *Patients, Medicine and the Law*, (2nd edn), Harmondsworth: Penguin.
British Medical Association (1993) *Medical Ethics Today: Its Practice and Philosophy*, London: BMA.
—— (1995) *Advance Statements About Medical Treatment*, London: BMA.
British Medical Association/Law Society (1995) *Assessment of Mental Capacity*, London: BMA/Law Society.
Brock, D. (1991) 'Trumping advance directives', *Hastings Center Report*, Supplement: S5–6.
—— (1993) 'A proposal for the use of advance directives in the treatment of incompetent mentally ill persons', *Bioethics*, 7 (2/3): 247–56.
Brock, D. and Buchanan, A. (1989) *Deciding For Others: The Ethics of Surrogate Decision Making*, Cambridge: Cambridge University Press.
Brown, J. *et al.* (1986) 'Is it normal for terminally ill patients to desire death?', *American Journal of Psychology*, 143: 208–11.
Cantor, N. (1993) *Advance Directives and the Pursuit of Death with Dignity*, Bloomington: Indiana University Press.
Chambers, C. *et al.* (1994) 'Relationship of advance directives to hospital charges in a medicare population', *Archives Internal Medicine*, 154: 541–7.
Cohen-Mansfield, J. *et al.* (1991) 'The decision to execute a durable power of attorney for health care and preferences regarding the utilization of life-sustaining treatments in nursing home residents', *Archives Internal Medicine*, 151: 289–94.
Cutter, M. and Shelp, E. (1991) *Competency: A Study of Informal Competency Determinations in Primary Care*, Dordrecht: Kluwer Academic Publishers.
Danis, M. *et al.* (1988) 'Patients' and families' preferences for medical intensive care', *Journal of American Medical Association*, 260: 797–802.
Danis, M. *et al.* (1991) 'A prospective study of advance directives for life-sustaining care', *New England Journal of Medicine*, 324: 882–8.
Davidson, K. and Moseley, R. (1989) 'Talking with patients about advance directives: the role of the primary care physician', in C. Hackler *et al.* (eds) *Advance Directives in Medicine*, New York: Praeger.
Dawson, A. (forthcoming) 'Arguments against advance directives'.
Diamond, E. *et al.* (1989) 'Decision-making ability and advance directive preferences in nursing home patients and proxies', *Gerontologist*, 29: 622–6.
Dillner, L. (1994) 'Relatives keener on euthanasia than patients', *British Medical Journal*, 309: 1107.
Doukas, D. and McCullough, L. (1991) 'The values history: the evaluation of the patient's values and advance directives', *Journal of Family Practice*, 32: 145–53.
Dresser, R. (1989) 'Advance directives, self-determination and personal identity', in C. Hackler *et al.* (eds) *Advance Directives in Medicine*, New York: Praeger.

Dworkin, R. (1993) *Life's Dominion: An Argument about Abortion and Euthanasia*, London: HarperCollins.

Eisendrath, S. and Jonsen, A. (1983) 'The living will', *Journal of American Medical Association*, 249(15): 2054–8.

Emanuel, E. and Emanuel, L. (1992) 'Proxy decision making for incompetent patients', *Journal of American Medical Association*, 267(15): 2067.

Emanuel, L. (1993) 'Advance directives: what have we learned so far?', *Journal of Clinical Ethics*, 4(1): 8–16.

Emanuel, L. and Emanuel, E. (1989) 'The medical directive: a new comprehensive advance care document', *Journal of American Medical Association*, 261: 3288–93.

Emanuel, L. *et al.* (1991a) 'Advance directives for medical care – a case for greater use', *New England Journal of Medicine*, 324(13): 889–95.

—— (1991b) 'Advance directives: how do scenario based treatment choices change over time?', *Clinical Research*, 40: 612A.

Epstein, A. (1989) 'Using proxies to evaluate quality of life: can they provide valid information about patients' health status and satisfaction with medical care?', *Medical Care*, 27 (Supp): S91–8.

Erin, C. and Harris, J. (1994) 'Living wills: anticipatory decisions and advance directives', *Reviews Clinical Gerontology*, 4: 269–75.

Everhart, M. and Perlman, R. (1990) 'Stability of patient preferences regarding life-sustaining treatments', *Chest*, 97: 159–64.

Faden, R. and Beauchamp, T. (1986) '*A History and Theory of Informed Consent*, New York: Oxford University Press.

Gamble, E. *et al.* (1991) 'Knowledge, attitudes and behaviour of elderly persons regarding living wills', *Archives Internal Medicine*, 151: 277–80.

Gibson, J. and Nathanson, P. (1990) 'The values history; an innovation in surrogate decision-making', *Law, Medicine and Health Care*, 18: 202–12.

Gillon, R. (1986) *Philosophical Medical Ethics*, Chichester: Wiley.

Government Response to the Report of the Select Committee on Medical Ethics (Cm 2553), HMSO, 1994.

Gutheil, T. and Appelbaum, P. (1983) 'Substituted judgement: best interests in disguise', *Hastings Center Report*, 13(3): 8–11.

Gunn, M. (1994) 'The meaning of incapacity', *Medical Law Review*, 2(1): 8–29.

Hackler, C., Moseley, R. and Vawter, D. (eds) (1989) *Advance Directives in Medicine*, New York: Praeger.

Heintz, L. (1988) 'Legislative hazard: keeping patients living, against their wills', *Journal of Medical Ethics*, 14: 82–6.

High, D. (1988) 'All in the family: extended autonomy and expectations in surrogate health care decision-making', *Gerontologist*, 28 (suppl): S46–51.

House of Lords (1994) *Report of the Select Committee on Medical Ethics. Volume 1: Report*, (HL Paper 21-I) HMSO.

Juengst, E. and Weil, C. (1989) 'Interpreting proxy directives: clinical decision-making and the durable power of attorney for health care', in C. Hackler, *et al.* (eds), *Advance Directives in Medicine*, New York: Praeger.

Kapp, M. (1982) 'Response to the living will furore: directives for maximum care', *American Journal of Medicine*, 72: 855–9.

Kass, L. (1980) 'Ethical dilemmas in the care of the ill', *Journal of American Medical Association*, 244: 1946.

Kennedy, I. and Grubb, A. (1994) *Medical Law: Text With Materials*, (2nd edn), London: Butterworths.

King, N. (1996) *Making Sense of Advance Directives*, Washington D.C.: Georgetown University Press.

Kutner, L. (1969) 'Due process of euthanasia: the living will, a proposal', *Indiana Law Journal*, 44: 539–54.

La Puma, J. *et al.* (1991) 'Advance directives on admission', *Journal of American Medical Association*, 266(3): 402–5.

La Puma, J. and Schiedermayer, D. (1991) 'The bookie, the girlfriend and the vultures; durable power of attorney complicated by financial conflict of interest', *Annals International Medicine*, 114: 98.

Law Commission (1995) *Law Commission Report No. 231: Mental Incapacity*, London: HMSO.

Lo, B. (1990) 'Assessing decision-making capacity', *Law, Medicine and Health Care*, 18(3): 193–201.

Lo, B. *et al.* (1986) 'Patient attitudes to discussing life-sustaining treatment', *Archives Internal Medicine*, 146: 1613–5.

Loewy, E. (1988) 'Changing one's mind: when is Odysseus to be believed?', *Journal General Internal Medicine*, 3: 54–8.

Loewy, E. and Carlson, R. (1994) 'Talking, advance directives, and medical practice', *Archives Internal Medicine*, 154: 2265–7.

Lord Chancellor's Department (1997) *Who Decides?: Making Decisions on Behalf of Mentally Incapacitated Adults*, London: The Stationery Office.

Luttrell, S. and Sommerville, A. (1996) 'Limiting risks by curtailing rights: a response to Dr Ryan', *Journal of Medical Ethics*, 22: 100–4.

Lynn, J. (1992) 'Procedures for making medical decisions for incompetent adults', *Journal of American Medical Association*, 267(15): 2082–4.

McLean, S. (ed.) (1996) *Death, Dying and the Law*, Aldershot: Dartmouth.

Magaziner, J. *et al.* (1988) 'Patient-proxy response comparability on measures of patient health and functional status', *Journal of Clinical Epidemiology*, 33: 1065–74.

Markson, L. *et al.* (1994) 'Implementing advance directives in the primary care setting', *Archives Internal Medicine*, 154: 2321–7.

Modell, W. (1974) 'A "will" to live', *New England Journal of Medicine*, 290(16): 907–8.

Montgomery, J. (1997) *Health Care Law*, Oxford: Oxford University Press.

Noonan, H. (1989) *Personal Identity*, London: Routledge.

Ouslander, J. *et al.* (1989) 'Health care decisions among elderly long-term care residents and their potential proxies', *Archives Internal Medicine*, 149: 1367–72.

Parfit, D. (1973) 'Later selves and moral principles', in A. Montefiore, (ed.) *Philosophy and Personal Relations*, London: Routledge & Kegan Paul.

Parfit, D. (1984) *Reasons and Persons*, Oxford: Oxford University Press.

Pellegrino, E. and Thomasma, D. (1988) *For the Patient's Good*, Oxford: Oxford University Press.

President's Commission (1982) *Making Health Care Decisions*, Washington D.C.: US GPO.

—— (1983) *Deciding to Forego Life-Sustaining Treatment*, Washington D.C.: US GPO.

Rosner, F. (1994) 'Living wills', *Lancet*, 343: 1041.

Rubenstein, L. (1984) 'Systematic biases in functional status assessment of elderly adults: effects of different data sources', *Journal of Gerontology*, 39: 686–91.

Ryan, C. (1996) 'Betting your life: an argument against certain advance directives', *Journal of Medical Ethics*, 22: 95–9.

Sachs, G. *et al.* (1990) 'Failure of an intervention to promote discussion of advance directives', *Journal American Geriatric Society*, 38(8): 3. Abstract.

Schlyter, C. (1992) *Advance Directives and AIDS*, London: Centre of Medical Law and Ethics, KCL.

Schneiderman, L. *et al.* (1990) 'Medical futility: its meaning and ethical implications', *Annals Internal Medicine*, 112: 949–54.

—— (1992) 'Effects of offering advance directives on medical treatment and costs', *Annals Internal Medicine*, 117: 599–606.

Seckler, A. *et al.* (1991) 'Substituted judgement: how accurate are proxy predictions', *Annals Internal Medicine*, 115: 92–8.

Sehgal, A. *et al.* (1992) 'How strictly do dialysis patients want their advance directives followed?', *Journal of American Medical Asociation*, 267: 59–63.

Silverman, H. *et al.* (1994) 'Nurses' perspectives on implementation of the PSDA', *Journal of Clinical Ethics*, 5(1): 30–7.

Silverstein, M. *et al.* (1991) 'Amyotrophic lateral sclerosis and life-sustaining therapy: patients' desires for information, participation in decision making and life-sustaining therapy', *Mayo Clinic Proceedings*, 66: 906–13.

Sommerville, A. (1996) 'Are Advance Directives Really the Answer?, in S. McLean (ed.) *Death, Dying and the Law*, Aldershot: Dartmouth.

Taranta, A. (1994) 'Living wills', *Lancet*, 343: 602.

Teno, J. *et al.* (1994) 'Do formal advance directives affect resuscitation decisions and the use of resources for seriously ill patients?', *Journal of Clinical Ethics*, 5(1): 23–30.

Thomasma, D. (1989) 'Advance directives and health care for the elderly', in Hackler *et al.* (eds) *Advance Directives in Medicine*, New York: Praeger.

Tomlinson, T. *et al.* (1990) 'An empirical study of proxy consent for elderly persons', *Gerontologist*, 29: 54–64.

Uhlmann, R. *et al.* (1988) 'Physicians' and spouses' predictions of elderly patients' resuscitation preferences', *Journal of Gerontology*, 43: M115–M121.

White, B. (1994) *Competence to Consent*, Washington D.C.: Georgetown University Press.

Wolf, S. *et al.* (1991) 'Sources of concern about the patient self-determination act', *New England Journal of Medicine*, 325(23): 1666–71.

Zweibel, N. and Cassel, C. (1989) 'Treatment choices at the end of life: a comparison of decisions by older patients and their physician-selected proxies', *Gerontologist*, 29: 615–21.

Chapter 10

The ethics of research in general practice

Roger Jones

INTRODUCTION

Research activity in primary care and community settings has increased greatly in recent years. The academic base of general practice has been consolidated as strong departments have grown up in the universities; there is now a chair of general practice in every medical school in the United Kingdom. As well as delivering an undergraduate medical curriculum, the university departments of general practice are active centres of multidisciplinary research in primary care.

The mid-1990s have also witnessed a heightened awareness of the importance of primary care within the National Health Service (NHS), and the concept of a 'primary care led NHS' has emerged. Linked to this have been explicit calls to strengthen and support research and development (R&D) activities in primary care and the community, and a funding mechanism for this was proposed in the Culyer Report (1996). The NHS R&D programme has also recognized the importance of research in primary care and a specific programme of work on research into the interface between primary and secondary care was commissioned in 1995/96 (Jones *et al.*, 1995). Further support for research in primary care has come from the recently-conducted Medical Research Council (MRC) topic review of research priorities in primary care. Finally, a national working party, set up by the NHS R&D programme, has considered mechanisms for increasing the research capacity of primary care, the training needs of primary care researchers and the most appropriate ways for universities, research councils, charities and the NHS to work together to strengthen the primary care research infrastructure (NHS Executive 1997). The Department of Health has made a commitment to doubling the R&D expenditure on primary care from approximately 7 per cent to 14 per cent over the next five years (Department of Health, 1996).

A number of specific ethical issues have emerged as research in the community and in general practice has expanded. Many of these are linked to the involvement in research of people in the community who are not themselves seeking medical care and to the potential impact of research on relationships between general practitioners and their patients, which traditionally are private and confidential and do not involve third party researchers.

In this chapter the ethical issues relevant to epidemiological, clinical trial and survey methodologies are identified and discussed. Many of the research methodologies involved in these studies are likely to be quantitative, but the recognition of the importance of qualitative research approaches also requires consideration. Qualitative studies are increasingly used to explore the beliefs, attitudes and perceptions of patients and professionals, to generate hypotheses which may be tested in subsequent quantitative work, to provide the thematic basis for questionnaire surveys and, in focus group work, to collect and synthesize views and information from groups as well as individuals (Britten *et al.*, 1996). This more 'personal' and potentially intrusive aspect of research generates substantial and often quite difficult ethical dilemmas.

RESEARCH IN GENERAL PRACTICE AND PRIMARY CARE

Background

The tradition of research in general practice can be traced back to the pioneering work of James MacKenzie and William Pickles through, in more recent years, John Fry, Julian Tudor Hart and John Howie, to the present day when general practice is part of a world-wide academic discipline, with a vigorous research and teaching culture (Jones, 1997).

Early research in general practice was usually descriptive. MacKenzie and Pickles, with remarkable foresight, were able to study the pattern, incidence and natural history of common conditions in the populations for which they were responsible. With the introduction of the National Health Service and patient registration, Fry was one of the first to capitalize on the unrivalled research opportunities presented by having an accurate population denominator, represented by the individual general practitioner's list of patients. For many years general practitioners operated a personal list system and were able to build up a detailed data set on a relatively small number, usually between 2–3,000, of patients.

The founding of the Royal College of General Practitioners and, in particular, their publication *Trends in General Practice* (Fry, 1977), set the scene for a research agenda which, with hindsight, developed along at least three parallel lines which, even today, are to some extent distinct and competitive. These are clinical research, health services research (which began with simple descriptions of the way that general practice is organized and the services delivered, but which has developed into a much more complex science evaluating service interventions) and the study of the relationship between general practitioners and their doctors. Whilst MacKenzie, Pickles and Fry could be regarded as the originators of a clinical research tradition, the study of the relationship between doctors and their patients began with the work of Michael Balint (1970), and has continued to represent a vigorous component of general practice research since the 1950s. Many authors have contributed to descriptions of the structures and processes of general practice and primary care, and this aspect of research has moved on from descriptive, survey methodologies to quasi-experimental and experimental techniques (Jones, 1997).

Research structures

When thinking about research in general practice it is often helpful to distinguish between research undertaken *by* general practitioners and other members of the primary care team, research *in* general practice and research *on* general practice. General practitioners, nurses, health visitors and managers may be involved in research concerning their own practice, but may also use general practice as a setting in which to examine other problems such as evaluation of drug therapies, studies on the natural history of common disorders and approaches to screening and health prevention. Research in general practice implies the involvement of general practitioners in data collection, but not necessarily in problem formulation. An extreme example of this approach is the Medical Research Council (MRC) general practice research framework, and many general practitioners are pleased to participate in multi-centre studies in which data collection represents the extent of their involvement in the research endeavour. Finally, research on general practice may be undertaken by a variety of individuals and specialists. A substantial proportion of publications in the *British Journal of General Practice* and, indeed, in the general practice section of the *British Medical Journal* are written by non-general practitioners. For example, studies on professional behavioural change are likely to involve contributions from medical sociologists and health psychologists, while evaluation of policy-led changes in general practice may be undertaken by health services researchers, health economists and others working in university departments or institutions other than those of general practice and primary care.

Research support

Research in general practice and community settings has, traditionally, been under-supported and under-funded, although the intellectual and policy tide has turned considerably in recent years. In the early days, the RCGP and the associated General Practice Research Club were important ways of providing support for otherwise isolated general practitioner researchers. As the university departments grew they were increasingly able to offer support for service GPs, but support structures, generally in the form of GP research networks, have become much more sophisticated in the last three to four years. Extensive and often well-funded GP research networks exist in many parts of the UK; examples include Noren, the northern research network, Wren, the Wessex research network, and STaRNet, the south Thames research network. Often funded through regional R&D budgets, these networks each involve large numbers (between 100–200) of general practitioners, with research skills and co-ordination being provided by specifically-appointed academic staff in the university departments of general practice associated with the network. The challenge for the future is to ensure that the funding mechanisms proposed by the Culyer Report (1996) enable adequate funds to flow from hospital settings into primary care to support this ever-growing research community (Jones *et al.*, 1995; NHS Executive, 1997).

Research funding for general practice has for many years been problematic. The RCGP, through its Scientific Foundation Board, was able to provide relatively small start-up research grants. Some regions had identified ear-marked research funds for primary care, but more often than not primary care researchers were in direct competition with projects from hospital and biomedical researchers whose proposals were, unsurprisingly, more comprehensible and probably more attractive to funding bodies. The MRC established a Health Services and Public Health Research Board to which researchers in primary care could apply for funding (although recent changes in the MRC funding arrangements may make this increasingly difficult).

The NHS R&D programme has, however, provided welcome and significant support for general practice-based research, not only in relation to the primary:secondary care interface, but also to the increasing recognition of evaluating interventions and treatments in the settings in which they were designed, rather than always relying on secondary care evaluations. Other significant sources of research funding for general practice include European Union programmes such as Biomed, Copernicus and Tempus, other medical charities in the UK and regional and health authority development funds. Departments of general practice are usually able to provide potential researchers with details of appropriate funding bodies and agencies.

Research outputs

Publication opportunities for general practice have also expanded in the last ten to fifteen years. The *British Journal of General Practice*, previously the *Journal of the Royal College of General Practitioners*, now has the highest impact factor of all primary care journals, and the *British Medical Journal* has a specific general practice section for original research papers. *Family Practice* was founded by Oxford University Press in conjunction with the RCGP twelve years ago, and is now a leading international journal of primary care. The *Scandinavian Journal of Primary Care*, *Family Medicine* in the United States and the recently-founded *European Journal of General Practice* also provide publication opportunities for primary care-based research. There are, however, many other journals in which research undertaken in and on general practice are published, including *Social Science and Medicine*, the *International Journal of Epidemiology*, *Quality and Health Care*, the *Journal of Health Service Policy and Research*, as well as more specialized journals devoted to specific clinical disciplines.

Dissemination and implementation of research findings has been recognized in recent years as being of the utmost importance; it is no longer safe to assume that research data appearing in a peer-reviewed journal will find their way into practice. Much research has been undertaken into the factors impacting on general practitioners' clinical behaviour, particularly in relation to research and educational interventions, and the NHS R&D programme has funded a programme of work on this topic. The ability to undertake critical appraisal of published material is now tested in the membership examination of the RCGP and the formation of general practice research networks around the country is also likely to contribute to a critical and evaluative culture. Evidence-based medicine has emerged as a catch phrase of the 1990s, with its own journal and culture.

The quality of research undertaken in general practice is of critical importance. We now have to compete on a level playing field for relatively scarce research funds and submit to peer assessment of research performance in the university sector. The continued funding of the community-based sciences in universities is critically dependent on research excellence, and the four yearly research assessment exercises cycle (RAE) undertaken by the Higher Education Funding Councils is of particular concern to the academic community. The methodologies used to assess research quality and determine the resource consequences of changes in these assessments include the quality of selected papers published by members of university departments, the size and origin of research grants attracted by them and the impact of the research themes and output of departments at national and international level. Success in the RAE is an important goal for senior academics in general practice and primary care.

THE ETHICAL BACKGROUND

Ethical principles

The ethical principles outlined by Gillon (1990) have been widely incorporated into undergraduate and postgraduate teaching about the ethics of modern medicine. Many of these principles, which are not discussed in detail in this chapter, are directly applicable to a consideration of the ethics of primary care research. Within Gillon's framework, respect of patients' autonomy and the pursuit of beneficence, non-maleficence and justice are regarded as cardinal ethical duties which apply with equal force to medical research.

It is, however, important to recognize that other approaches to the ethics of medicine and medical research may contribute to the solution of problems generated by research in community settings. Seedhouse's (1988) notion that 'work for health is a moral endeavour' has some appeal, with its implications that the research aspect of 'medical work' should, likewise, represent a moral endeavour, the outcomes of which should include enhancing the potential and well being of individuals. The 'ethical grid' proposed by Seedhouse begins with the fundamental requirement of respect for individuals. The creation and respect of autonomy and the requirement to meet needs before wants are also essentials in Seedhouse's system. At the next level in the grid the minimization of harm, truth-telling, promise-keeping and an intention to enable (Seedhouse's equivalent of beneficence) are of central importance.

We work and live in a multi-cultural society, and it may be that we have to be prepared to explore and grapple with ethical and moral views held by other cultures which may not always be directly compatible with the essentially Judaeo-Christian ethical framework of traditional medicine and medical research. There is a large and growing literature on medical ethics and, as biomedicine meets increasingly difficult therapeutic challenges, issues of consent and confidentiality and equipoise in the conduct of randomized controlled trials, for instance, may assume increasing significance (Freedman, 1994).

Problems in practice

From an NHS point of view perhaps the most important background characteristic of general practice research is that the surgery, the health centre and the community are not traditional settings for undertaking research. Patients are likely to be unfamiliar with the concept of research under these circumstances and the majority of them will not be familiar with the increasing use of general practice as a teaching setting. Ethical problems may arise in the recruitment and involvement of individuals who are not seeking medical care and in the relationships among them, patients in the surgery, their general practitioners and the researchers or research team, who may themselves be general practitioners.

Autonomy will always be threatened, and may be compromised, when individuals are requested to participate in research studies. In the United Kingdom, Norway and the Netherlands, general practitioners now hold lists of patients registered with them, including demographic details of individual patients. It is possible to search these databases so that information about age, sex, morbidity, prescribing and other factors can all be extracted by the use of computer software. This means that general practice registers are increasingly accessible and, therefore, attractive as sampling frames for epidemiological and community-based research, particularly for studies concerned with people in the community who have not yet entered medical care.

Individuals can be identified and selected from databases of this kind and requested to participate in data collection either through postal questionnaires or interviews. These patients, however, have provided personal information for the purpose of obtaining clinical care, not for research purposes; for their general practitioner to disclose such information to researchers, without permission, could be construed as breaking medical confidentiality, threatening patient autonomy and could have legal consequences. It would, of course, be possible for general practitioners to request permission from individual patients before granting researchers access to their names and addresses, identifying them as members of a particular diagnostic category or, for that matter, approaching them themselves for their own research purposes. These procedures, however, are likely to add substantially to the time and costs involved in undertaking the research, particularly in large-scale epidemiological work when information on several thousand subjects may be required. These workload implications may also make general practitioners reluctant to participate in research initiated elsewhere. It might, on the other hand, be argued that the simple act of supplying researchers with a list of names and addresses does not compromise patient confidentiality as long as no other information is released. This view would facilitate population-based studies, but further problems will arise in relation to sending reminders to non-respondents which evidently involved disclosure of patients' personal details to the researchers. Decisions about the appropriateness of seeking prior consent will clearly relate to the nature of the information divulged, the research methods proposed and the scale of the study being undertaken and will need to be made after close consultation between the research group and the general practitioners involved.

Whether or not patients' permission is obtained before access to these databases is granted, general practitioners should always be provided with a list of potential participants in studies so that this can be scrutinized to ensure that those unsuitable, either for medical or personal reasons, are excluded from sampling and are not approached by the researchers. Clearly, however, this approach is a potential source of bias; general practitioners may feel protective about certain patients, may not wish personal acquaintances to be involved in research or may have other reasons for excluding certain subjects from research studies.

Problems for patients

When patients are selected to participate in a research study, even if they are not concerned about the disclosure of their medical details, anxiety may be provoked by the invitation to participate. Patients are often surprised at being included in surveys and may have difficulty in dealing with the concept of random selection. They may fear that their selection for research on a clinical topic indicates that their general practitioner or the research group is in possession of information about them of which they themselves are unaware. In studies employing quota or stratified sampling this may, naturally, be a correct interpretation, because patients will have been selected precisely because they have certain medical or other characteristics. It is very important to try to deal with these problems by describing to subjects the information that has been made available to the researchers and clarifying not only the reason for their selection but the method used to select them.

There is a potential conflict between ensuring that patients feel at liberty to decline to participate in research on the one hand and, on the other, maximizing response rates. One approach that is used widely to maximize response rates is the use of personalized and explanatory leaflets from general practitioners, using practice letterheads and a personal approach to patients and emphasizing the importance of the study and urging co-operation in completing questionnaires or attending an interview. Under these circumstances patients may quite understandably feel reluctant to refuse, either because of personal loyalty to the general practitioner concerned or simply because they think that they may be discriminated against in the future provision of medical care. Although this is usually a successful strategy in optimizing response rates to requests to participate in research, it is certainly at least potentially coercive. One possible solution is for patients to be assured that their general practitioner will not be informed about whether or not they have taken part in the study and that future care will not be compromised, but it is difficult to include both assurances in the same letter.

When we write to patients assuring them that information collected in the course of research will be anonymous and confidential, these words need careful consideration before we can use them with conviction and accuracy. It may be preferable to use other words such as non-attributable, because the act of sending a reminder letter negates the notion of anonymity, and the sharing of information about individuals with researchers makes the use of 'confidentiality' in its strict sense difficult.

The concept of informed consent in the setting of access to patients' databases and records assumes that patients have adequate information upon which to base their decisions about participation. This, however, is not a straightforward issue because a competence gap involving knowledge and understanding is likely to exist between biomedical and social researchers and many of their subjects. For example, researchers may, for the sake of clarity, over-simplify the research project to which they hope to recruit subjects, and they need to be careful not to use this process of simplification to obscure the true nature and details of the research.

It is important for researchers to provide a clear explanation to subjects and patients about what is likely to be involved if they agree to take part in the research, and to be as clear as they can about the likely time commitment and the possible inconvenience, risks and discomfort entailed. Patient information leaflets, accompanying invitations to participate in research, may be helpful. In questionnaire surveys it is not unusual to ask whether the subject is prepared to be contacted again by the researchers; the nature of this contact is often not specified and may well result in a request for an in-depth interview, which may be conducted in the patient's home. If the patient was unaware of this eventuality, they may find themselves in a difficult position. Although patients are free to decline to participate at a later date, it is more helpful to give them information about the nature of the proposed follow-up at the recruitment stage.

The consultation

Recruitment of patients for research studies may also take place at their point of contact with the health care system, either on entering the surgery premises, where they may be presented with a questionnaire on registration at the reception desk, in the waiting room, where they may similarly be given research documentation, or in the consulting room itself. All of these situations are potentially coercive for patients, but a request to take part in research made in the course of a routine consultation may be the most difficult of all. Patients will have made the decision to consult, which itself may not have been easy to do, in the entirely reasonable belief that the whole encounter will be confidential. The possibility that their reasons for seeking health care may become open to scrutiny is likely to be anxiety-provoking.

There are a number of approaches which preserve autonomy and reduce the chances of causing harm. Patients should certainly be given a 'cooling off' period, analogous to that applied to some financial agreements, before agreeing to participate in a research study when the invitation was made in the surgery setting. Written consent from patients is usually needed when patients are recruited by these methods, although being approached in the surgery for an interview, or even being asked to complete a questionnaire, may be more difficult to safeguard.

Patients consult their general practitioners believing that everything that happens in the consultation will be confidential, yet the consultation itself may act as a trigger for involvement in the research study. The general practitioner may ask the patient directly if they will be prepared to participate in, for example, a randomized controlled trial of a treatment intervention or the general practitioner's referral letter to a hospital specialist might act as a trigger for involvement. If the aim of the research study is to observe general practitioner referral behaviour, for example, the general practitioner concerned may be unaware of the inclusion of a specific patient in the study and, therefore, will not be able to ask the patient for consent to participate. One possible consequence of this could be that the patient then receives a research questionnaire even before they have heard from the hospital appointments office to see the specialist. This is embarrassing and unsatisfactory, and study design should take account of these potential pitfalls. Other clinical events such as writing a prescription or arranging an investigation may also act as triggers for inclusion in research and it is important that patients know that a study is underway and that they are at risk of being included in it, even if the precise method of patient selection is not clear to the medical professional concerned. All of these triggers for involvement in research raise questions about the confidentiality of the encounter between a patient and a health care professional and the status of patient autonomy.

DATA COLLECTION

Quantitative methods

Epidemiological studies may give rise to particular problems about the ethical responsibilities of researchers in relation to dealing with the information collected, often using questionnaires, from large numbers of patients. One example is a study that set out to document the prevalence of gastrointestinal symptoms in the community. Because of the large sample required to obtain the necessary precision in the study, a small proportion of subjects turned out to have a complex of symptoms suggesting the possibility of serious, but hitherto unrecognized, gastrointestinal disease (Jones and Tait, 1995). These symptoms included rectal bleeding, changes in bowel habit, persistent abdominal pain, weight loss and difficulty in swallowing, and were reported by patients responding to structured questionnaires designed to determine the prevalence of such symptoms. The patients had been selected at random from registers held by health authorities and the general practitioners had carefully vetted the lists of participating patients before contact by post. What are the ethical obligations of the research team to their patients and to their general practitioners in terms of beneficence, non-maleficence and autonomy?

The individual general practitioners involved in this study expressed an interesting range of views. Some insisted that information of this kind should be reported immediately so that appropriate action, perhaps an invitation for the registered patient to consult their general practitioner, might be taken (Crosland and Jones, 1995). This, clearly, could be construed as a breach of the confidentiality and anonymity promised by the researchers, even when such reporting is likely to have been in the medical interests of the patient concerned. Autonomy is in conflict with beneficence. Some doctors, however, took an entirely opposite ethical stance, and asserted that patients have a right to make their own decisions about whether or not to consult. Although this position can to some extent be countered by arguing that many individuals simply do not have enough specialized information on which to base an informed decision about seeking medical advice, its proponents argued that patient autonomy and confidentiality of information should have taken precedence over uninvited medical intervention.

This situation can be further complicated when the epidemiological survey represents part of a longer-term study to determine the course and natural history of a disease. Subsequent observations may be distorted if patients have been subjected to therapeutic interventions or have been removed altogether from the study because of the recognition of the significance of symptoms in the first data set. It is essential that these issues are discussed and resolved to the satisfaction of the research team, the participating general practitioners and the subjects of the research before the research begins.

Structured questionnaires may be administered by interviewers to obtain information in health care or domestic settings, and raise rather different questions. For example respondents are usually given a restricted choice of acceptable answers and they may be asked to reduce complicated thinking about difficult issues to a set of ticked boxes. Patients may find this an anonymous and unnerving experience, particularly if they are talking about emotionally significant issues. Interviewers are likely to have been instructed to adopt a neutral manner in the search for reliability and this again can de-personalize the encounter, perhaps leaving patients feeling exploited.

As a minimum interviewers should establish a more symmetrical relationship with the interviewee before the interview starts, and allow time for debriefing after completion of the questionnaire. It may, for example, be worth offering patients the opportunity at the end of the interview to communicate more of the complexity of their experience, and consideration could be given to the inclusion of free-text and narrative responses in the questionnaire, even if these cannot necessarily be used in subsequent analysis.

Qualitative studies

When seeking more complex information through in-depth interviews, the opposite problems to those raised by structured questionnaires may be encountered, particularly in relation to the interaction between the subject and the interviewer. Careful listening by a trained and skilled interviewer can be a therapeutic experience; for most of us it is unusual to be listened to with sympathy and without interruption. This means that subjects taking part in these interviews can become more aware than usual of distressing emotions or life difficulties which, for the rest of the time, they might be able to ignore. Although acknowledging this distress is not in itself damaging, it does raise the question of how it can be dealt with by the interviewer. The interviewer may feel that it is impossible to leave the subject at the end of an interview, and may attempt to stay in contact to try to help the subject cope with the distress disclosed. Clearly it is impossible to maintain contact with everyone who is interviewed and interviewers need to recognize that the subjects who have agreed to be interviewed did so on the understanding that this was not going to be a long-term therapeutic relationship. One solution is to schedule a second interview to debrief the subject and help the subject deal with the distress in studies in which difficult material has been elicited and a significant emotional impact may be anticipated.

There may, however, be disadvantages in this approach; the very transience of the interviewer–subject relationship may generate a safe environment in which subjects may be much more frank and open than they otherwise would. They can take risks, knowing that there will be no follow-up; remaining in contact would not allow such uninhibited disclosure.

Interviewees may, however, disclose other facets of their illnesses that are unknown to their general practitioners. This poses considerable difficulties, similar to those discussed in relation to epidemiological studies, in which medical information is presented to a researcher (the interviewer) who may not have the medical knowledge and expertise to evaluate its significance. Unfortunately the subject may assume that the interviewer is in fact able to understand the significance of this information, possesses medical expertise and contacts and that they will act appropriately in the subject's interest. It is conceivable that the subject will assume that the interviewer will pass the information on to the general practitioner concerned. Clear communication with interviewees about these issues is important so that confusion and misunderstanding can be avoided; interviewers need to be explicit about the extent to which they are able to respond to medical information provided by interviewees or are willing or able to pass this information on to appropriate medical professionals.

A number of methodological and ethical issues arise in participant observation studies, which are increasingly used in general practice and might include the use of simulated patients or the direct observation of patient–professional interactions. Most of these problems relate to the principle of informed consent; in some participant observation studies those being observed need to be kept in ignorance of the presence or intentions of the researcher, such as general practitioners dealing with simulated patients in their surgeries. This research does, of course, have significant methodological advantages because it minimizes bias and reactivity, the risk that the findings are an artefact of the research process itself. Negotiating permission to undertake research of this kind is clearly of great importance, but there is a danger that the researchers will negotiate with the more powerful members of the medical group, generally doctors, but not with the less influential members, such as nurses, receptionists, secretarial staff and patients. Furthermore, it is simply not practicable to negotiate access with everybody concerned, particularly if observations are being made of activities in an open or public place such as a health centre waiting room or reception area. Nonetheless, the confidentiality and autonomy of those concerned in work of this kind should be respected and safeguarded as far as possible by the use of written information where appropriate and verbal discussion and notification in other circumstances.

GENERAL ETHICAL ISSUES

Confidentiality, anonymity and non-attribution are important in relation to patient consent for quantitative research methodologies, but it may be very difficult, if not impossible, to obscure the identity of the setting in which research is being carried out. This may be particularly important in qualitative work; practice team members could recognize themselves and each other in the description of a practice, for example. When narrative material is quoted directly in research papers, anonymity may be preserved but confidentiality is of necessity abandoned. Researchers should give some thought to the kind of reports and publications likely to be generated by their research studies, and it might be appropriate under certain circumstances to discuss this with subjects in advance of interviews or other contacts. Seeing one's own statements in print, either as a professional or a lay person, can only serve to undermine earlier assurances of confidentiality, which may have been given injudiciously.

The possibility that sinister medical information may emerge in the course of research has already been mentioned, particularly in relation to beneficence and non-maleficence, but it is also important to recognize the need for clear ground rules for non-medical researchers in dealing with sensitive or alarming information revealed by patients. This is a difficult practical problem, because a strong feeling of empathy is likely to emerge in the course of a lengthy interview; researchers should not be drawn into giving opinions, but may become anxious when patients describe something which sounds as if it should be clinically investigated. There may, for example, be situations where disclosure should take precedence over confidentiality, as discussed earlier, but consideration also needs to be given to the legal implications for the researcher of non-disclosure of information. In some situations the consent form may include a legal disclaimer. For example, a non-consulting subject with rectal bleeding and changed bowel habit, reported at interview to a non-medical researcher, might justifiably feel aggrieved when, at a later date, disseminated colorectal cancer is diagnosed.

Other information disclosed at interview may also give rise to problems; research in areas such as child abuse may create difficult ethical dilemmas for researchers who discover previously undisclosed activities, with inevitable conflicts between assurances of confidentiality and moral, and possibly legal, responsibilities to the children concerned. Another area which can create problems is that in which distress itself is the subject of research, such as individuals' responses to bereavement or terminal illness. The researcher may, under these circumstances, feel almost voyeuristic in the research and analysis of the distress of others.

Finally, an important issue for researchers undertaking qualitative research work in patients own homes is their own safety. Not only is it difficult to know in advance whether it will be 'safe' to interview a particular subject from the study, but some subjects may be selected for study on the very grounds that may call into question the safety of the interviewer, such as mental health, personality disorder or substance abuse. It is important that, particularly if travelling alone, interviewers ensure that colleagues in their department or place of work are aware of their destination, and their expected time of return. The use of pagers and mobile telephones may add to the sense of safety and security, and interviewers should feel free to discontinue interviews if, for whatever reason, the atmosphere becomes uncomfortable or threatening. These are ethical issues of particular relevance to directors of research, who must ensure that their researchers are treated with the same consideration as their research subjects (Jones *et al.*, 1995).

Dissemination of Research Results

Protecting the sources of research information is important and is part of the undertaking of confidentiality and anonymity. It may, however, be that going to excessive lengths to conceal the sources of data makes it impossible for readers of the research report fully to appreciate the setting in which the research was conducted and to determine whether the results can be generalized to their own setting. Outsiders may not recognize individuals or places, but insiders (the subject of the research) almost certainly will, and it is likely to be important for them to be able to see the research report before it is published.

Providing feedback to subjects may also be important in epidemiological studies. In one study on general practitioner referrals of patients with rectal bleeding, for example, 83 per cent of patients indicated that they would appreciate a copy of the report. In a qualitative study on patients' consulting behaviour, almost two-thirds of participants requested information about the results. This may indicate a wish for more involvement and information by subjects in some areas of research at least, although there are logistic difficulties in providing this information and also some problems of interpretation when the information forms part of a professional report. Clearly an abbreviated or summary version of the research can be produced separately.

The consequences of dissemination of research information for the participants also needs to be considered. Collecting information about, for example, smoking and drinking habits might simply stigmatize certain social groups and reinforce inappropriate stereotypes. Re-interpretation of research data because of the interests of the lay media may caricature not only the research findings but also the research subjects. Research that has implications for increasing the provision of medical services, with resource allocation implications, may create inappropriate expectations in the minds of the subjects and generate subsequent disappointments. Researchers also need to remember that future research collaboration is likely to be important, and the presentation and discussion of information in which criticism of the subjects of research is either explicit or implicit may jeopardize this.

Finally, it is important to consider the possibility of over-researching particular groups or individuals. It will be helpful for researchers to keep careful records of patients who have been approached to participate in studies, and for practices to do the same. This represents a further reason why general practitioners should always see lists of patients selected from registers before they are used for research purposes.

Research Ethics Committees

Researchers and their collaborators need to pay attention to the range of ethical issues involved in primary care research described above in the preparation of their research protocols. An additional safeguard is provided by the Research Ethics Committees (RECs) which are independent committees appointed by health authorities according to nationally-agreed guidelines. The committee has appointed members of both sexes, including a chair, deputy chair (s), a senior academic, medical members including at least one with expertise in general practice, lay and nursing members, a legal member and an administrator. The constitution aims to provide a balance of medical and non-medical representation. The chair and members are generally appointed for a specific period, generally three years renewable, and renewal depends on maintaining a membership with a wide range of specialist knowledge in relevant fields, including psychiatry, social science and research methodologies.

The RECs generally meet monthly, and a standard application form is completed and submitted in time for the next meeting. RECs are generally able to provide ethical approval either on the basis of the chair's action, either alone or after consultation with other committee members, or in committee, to which the researcher (s) may be invited. This determination will be based on the scientific validity of the research proposal and protocol, the way in which the research will be conducted, arrangements for informed consent and specific arrangements, where appropriate, including research on unconscious subjects, minors and research involving special risks.

The committee's approval is granted to specific investigators, who are responsible for notifying the committee of any ethical problems arising during the course of the project or any changes to the research protocol, and are responsible for providing a brief report after completion of the research. The committee will remind researchers that all records of research on human subjects must be kept securely for a minimum period of ten years.

The increasing standardization of the methods of working and the constitution of RECs is welcome. A number of publications have demonstrated a wide variation in the workload, methods of working, frequency of meeting and decision making of these committees, which may be particularly undesirable in the case of multi-centre studies (Foster, 1995). To further facilitate studies taking place on more than one site, many local RECs have agreed reciprocity of approval within defined geographical areas. A new system of Multicentre Research Ethics Committees (MRECs) has recently been introduced to deal specifically with multi-centre research studies.

CONCLUSIONS

Research in primary care generates a set of ethical questions, and some dilemmas, distinct from much of biomedical and clinical trials research. In particular, researchers in primary care have to be quite clear about their responsibilities to people in the community who have not yet sought or entered formal medical care and to patients registering and consulting with general practitioners who are doing so in the reasonable expectation of complete confidentiality and do not regard themselves at risk of being involved in research studies.

Little information is currently available about patients' views of being involved in research of this kind. This would be an important starting point for evaluating methods of making contact, providing information and consent and conducting research in these potentially vulnerable groups of patients.

Finally, teaching medical ethics and law in the undergraduate curriculum needs to include an account of the particular ethical questions raised by research taking place outside the traditional teaching hospital setting.

REFERENCES

Balint, M. (1970) *The Doctor, His Patient and the Illness*, London: Pitman Medical.

Britten, N., Jones, R., Murphy, E. and Stacy, R. (1996) 'Qualitative research methods in general practice and primary care', *Family Practice*, 12: 104–14.

Crosland, A. and Jones, R. (1995) 'Rectal bleeding in the community: prevalence and consultation behaviour', *British Medical Journal*, 311: 486–8.

Culyer Report (1996) *The New Funding System for Research and Development in the NHS*, London: Department of Health.

Department of Health (1996) *Primary Care: Delivering the Future*, London: HMSO.

Foster, C. (1995) 'Why do research ethics committees disagree with each other?', *Journal of Royal College of Physicians*, 29: 315–18.

Freedman, B. (1994) 'Equipoise and the ethics of clinical research', in T.L. Beauchamp and L. Walters Belmont (eds) *Contemporary Issues in Bioethics*, California: Wadsworth.

Fry, J. (ed.) (1977) *Trends in General Practice*, London: Royal College of General Practitioners.

Gillon, R. (1990) *Philosophical Medical Ethics*, Bristol: Wiley.

Jones, R. (1997) 'A liberal education: teaching, learning and research in general practice', *British Journal of General Practice*, 47: 395–9.
Jones, R. and Tait, C. (1995) 'Gastrointestinal side effects of nonsteroidal anti-inflammatory drugs in the community', *British Journal of Clinical Practice*, 49, 67–70.
Jones, R., Lamont, T. and Haines, A. (1995) 'Setting priorities for research and development in the NHS: a case study on the interface between primary and secondary care', *British Medical Journal*, 311: 1076–80.
Jones, R., Murphy, E. and Crosland, A. (1995) 'Primary care research ethics', *British Journal of General Practice*, 45: 623–6.
National Working Group on R&D in Primary Care (1996) *Delivering the Future*, London: HMSO.
NHS Executive (1997) *Final Report of the National Working Party in R&D in Primary Care*, Bristol: NHSE.
Seedhouse, D. (1988) *Ethics: The Heart of Medicine*, Chichester: Wiley.

Index

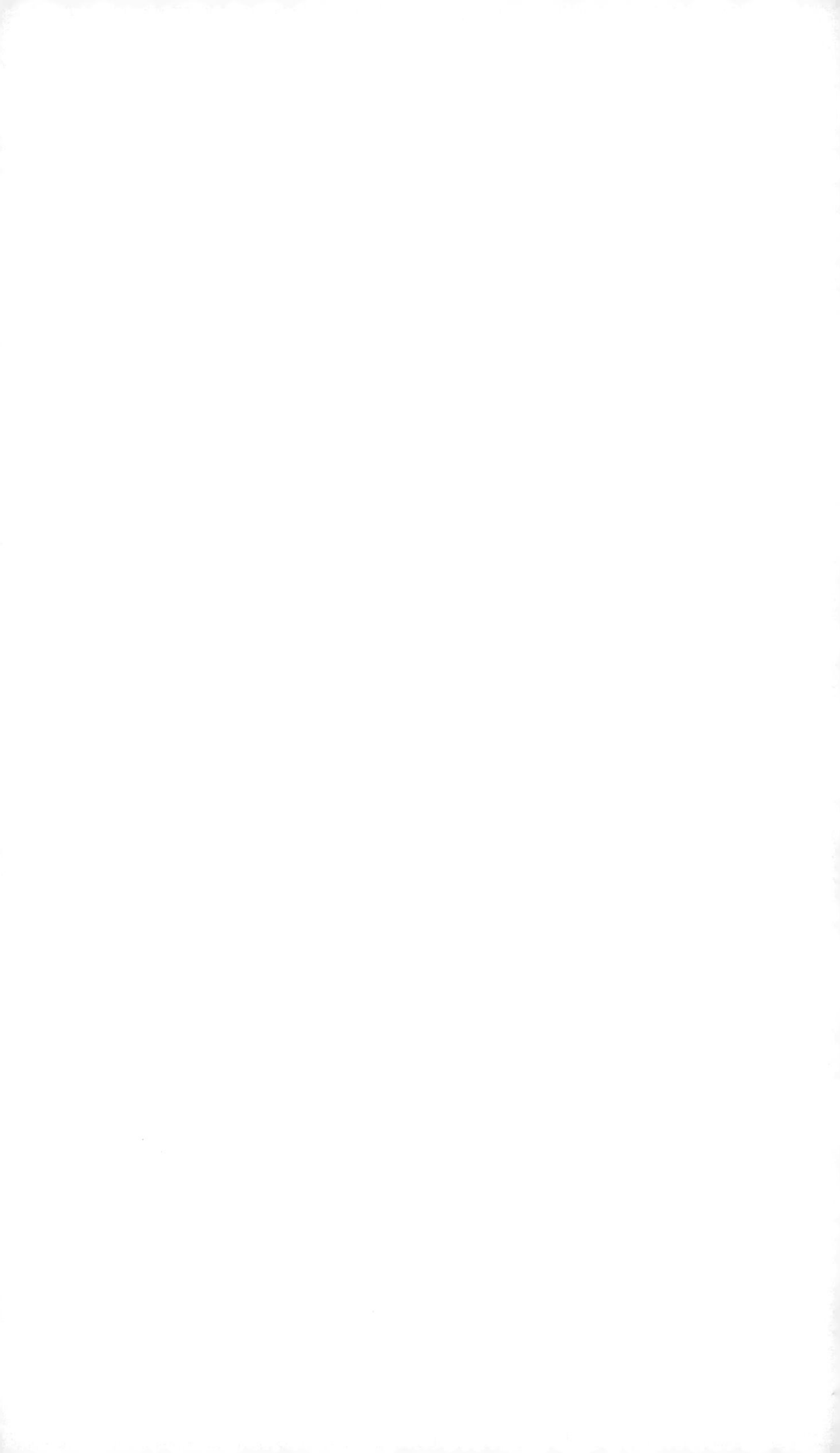

For Product Safety Concerns and Information please contact our EU
representative GPSR@taylorandfrancis.com
Taylor & Francis Verlag GmbH, Kaufingerstraße 24, 80331 München, Germany

www.ingramcontent.com/pod-product-compliance
Ingram Content Group UK Ltd.
Pitfield, Milton Keynes, MK11 3LW, UK
UKHW010813080625
459435UK00006B/58

* 9 7 8 0 4 1 5 1 6 4 9 9 3 *